Multiple Choice Questions in Optometry

Multiple Choice Questions in Optometry

R. Fletcher MSc(Tech) DCLP Dorth FBCO

Emeritus Professor of Optometry and Visual Science,
City University, London, UK

K.M. Oliver BSc(Hons) MBCO

Lecturer (some-time), Kongsberg College of
Engineering, Norway;
Researcher, Caledonian University, Glasgow, UK

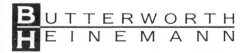

Butterworth-Heinemann Ltd
Linacre House, Jordan Hill, Oxford OX2 8DP

 A member of the Reed Elsevier plc group

OXFORD LONDON BOSTON
MUNICH NEW DELHI SINGAPORE SYDNEY
TOKYO TORONTO WELLINGTON

First published 1996

British Library Cataloguing in Publication Data
A catalogue record for this book is available from the British Library.

ISBN 0 7506 2187 7

Library of Congress Cataloguing in Publication Data
A catalogue record for this book is available from the Library of Congress.

Composition by Genesis Typesetting, Laser Quay, Rochester, Kent
Printed and bound in Great Britain by Biddles Ltd, Guildford and King's Lynn

Contents

Preface

The authors' varied experience in optometric practice includes contact with students at different levels and in different lands; both were educated in the British tradition of university-based optometric courses and have acted as examiners in different situations.

Multiple choice questions (MCQs) are popular in many professional examinations and very useful for revision. Candidates must develop some MCQ technique, not in order to be able to spot likely topics but rather to become familiar with the limited variety of approaches by which a correct, or most correct, response is needed. The time element is important in such examinations and practice helps towards quicker evaluation. There is some informed opinion that the MCQ is *most* valuable as an aid to learning and revision, whatever the merits as part of an examination.

A simple figure often replaces many words, giving examiners (in a non-MCQ context) extra and rapid insight into what a candidate wishes to express. A few sketches are given in this text as examples.

The preferred solution to each question is indicated on a separate page, usually with concise comments and some reference suggestions. Most sources are readily available as recent or classical textbooks, products of both sides of the Atlantic, plus some journal references.

Unfortunately the best answer to some questions can be a matter of opinion. One of the authors once gave answer 'A' to a first oral examiner's question, only to be told that the answer was absurd and that answer 'B' had been expected. Immediately afterwards in another room a second examiner asked virtually the same question; when answer B was timidly advanced as a possibility, the irate examiner indicated that answer A should have been produced as the only satisfactory response. It took some wriggling and elaboration to retrieve the situation. Actually, the examination was passed! We wish readers similar success and hope that this book will help.

How to use this text

Several subject groups have been used, with questions usually arranged in order of increasing difficulty. Readers should attempt all questions, even those that they might feel they have 'left behind'. Sometimes elementary matters may have to be faced in examinations, since they form the basis of later work.

Note how the text does not always use the preferred approach of particular examinations. The simple recall of facts is often needed but some questions demand the best solution for a relatively involved problem. You may have to evaluate data or to make (mental) calculations. The essential requirement is usually for the *choice* of the correct, best, or optimum alternative; sometimes you must find an incorrect statement.

Even if your answers are correct the first time, wait a few days and retest yourself.

The references involve textbooks and journals, most of which can be sought through good libraries and it is usually worthwhile taking the trouble to look up a high proportion; even if you have the correct answer, you may benefit from information as to why the false, or diversionary, suggestions were incorrect.

Do not neglect older journals and books, when recommended. Some basic facts do not alter and often the older material is easily located. But beware of changing attitudes. There was the optometrist who, years after ending his course, visited his old teacher and found him marking the latest examination. With some surprise he noted that the questions were the same as he had faced many years before. The teacher explained that he used the same questions, since patients' needs seldom varied. But he added, 'I change the answers, when necessary!' In fact, even some answers stand the test of time.

Students and optometrists outside the UK, can use this text as another way to understand the English language approach to a wide spectrum of professional knowledge. It should be helpful for those interested in a 'European Diploma of Optometry' or contemplating study in the UK.

The authors would welcome comment and suggestions, realizing as they do that the MCQ is a fruitful challenge to universal agreement.

R. Fletcher
K.M. Oliver

1 Visual optics

1 Keratometers can be used to measure convex (or concave) surfaces but their scales are limited to relatively normal 'corneal' radii. You wish to measure a spherical convex mirror of radius about 14 mm and so have to fix on to the instrument's objective an auxiliary spectacle lens. Which power of lens is most likely to be suitable?

A   −2.00 DS
B   +2.00 DS
C   +2.00 DS/−2.00 DC
D   +8.00 DS
E   −8.00 DS

2 The fibres of the crystalline lens sometimes enable a subject to observe 'physiological haloes' around a spot of light in darkness. Which of the following suggestions is most correct?

A   The orange–red extreme edge subtends about 9.5 degrees at the eye
B   The physiological halo tends to behave as rotating sectors when a stenopaeic slit is moved slowly across the pupil, in a direction at 90 degrees to the length of the slit, as in Figure 1.1
C   Such physiological haloes are of the same angular subtense as glaucoma haloes
D   Physiological haloes are about half the size of glaucoma haloes

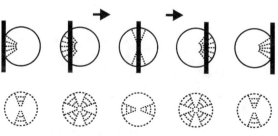

Fig. 1.1 Subjective appearances of haloes as slit passes across pupil.

1 Visual optics: Answers

1 Power A is best. A relatively low powered negative sphere permits the working distance of the instrument to increase and the image seen is smaller. A recalibration is needed, using surfaces of known curvature; the calibration for a concave surface would be different. An astigmatic lens is inappropriate as it would dictate the careful choice of a particular meridian suitable to its principal meridians and those of the instrument; it would mimic a toroidal surface.

References

Douthwaite, W.A. (1987) *Contact Lens Optics*, Butterworths, London, pp. 77 and 146

Emsley, H.H. *Visual Optics*, various edns, Hatton Press, London (see index of each edition)

Fletcher, R., Lupelli, L. and Rossi, A. (1994) *Contact Lens Practice*, Blackwell Scientific, Oxford, p. 124

Phillips, A.J. and Stone, J. (1989) *Contact Lenses*, 3rd edn, Butterworths, London, p. 248

Quesnel, N.M. and Simonet, P. (1994) Precision and reliability study of a modified keratometric technique for measuring the radius of curvature of soft contact lenses. *Ophthal Physiol Opt*, **14**, 320–325 (regarding a Zeiss instrument and some novel aspects)

2 B is the only correct description. While glaucoma haloes are about 9 degrees in size and relatively bright, physiological haloes caused by lens fibres are only a little smaller, while the transitory physiological haloes attributable to corneal mucus drops tend to be larger. It is the exposure of differently orientated lens fibres by changes in the slit's position which produce the effect of rotation.

References

Bennett, A. G. and Rabbetts, R.B. (1989) *Clinical Visual Optics*, 2nd edn, Butterworths, London, pp. 507–508

Brown, F.G. and Fletcher, R. (1990) *Glaucoma in Optometric Practice*, Blackwell Scientific, Oxford, pp. 63–66

Elliot, R.H. (1924) A halometer. *Brit Med J*, 5 April

Emsley, H.H. and Fincham, E.F. (1921–22) Diffraction halos in normal and glaucomatous eyes. *Trans Opt Soc* XXIII, **4**(15), 225

Heilmann, K. and Richardson, K.T., eds (1978) *Glaucoma, Conceptions of a Disease*, Saunders, Philadelphia, p. 151 (for another sort of glaucoma halo, observed ophthalmoscopically!)

Hoskins, H.D. and Kass, M.A. (1989) *Diagnosis and Therapy of the Glaucomas*, Mosby, St Louis, p.9.

3 Patients with partial sight can benefit from advice as to the optimum use of a *loupe* or magnifier which is fixed in a stand. Take the example of an emmetrope using a +20 DS (assumed to be thin) for reading newsprint which is fixed at 4 cm from the lens (Figure 1.2). Decide which of the following items is most likely to be true. (Any calculations needed should be possible mentally or on scrap paper.)

A Least accommodation would be needed if the eye were very close to the lens

B Approximately 3 D of accommodation would be needed if the eye were to be about 13.33 cm from the lens

C The field of view would be greatest with the eye as far from the lens as possible

D The magnification would be independent of the distance between lens and eye

E The amount of accommodation required does not depend on the distance between the newsprint and the lens

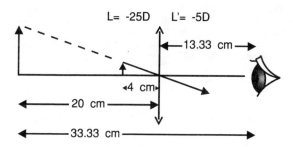

Fig. 1.2 Ray diagram of magnifier in use.

3   B is correct, since the lens presents to the eye a virtual image
20 cm behind the lens. Thus an eye in contact with the lens
requires 5 D and an eye 13.33 cm from the lens requires only 3 D
of accommodation. The simple diagram impresses this
comparison. Presumably a spectacle addition could be used
instead of accommodation. If the Sloan system of magnification
(referred to a nominal distance of 40 cm) is used so that

$$M_{40} = \frac{\text{Lens power} + \text{acc.} - (d \times \text{acc.} \times \text{lens power})}{2.5}$$

(where d is vertex distance in metres), in one case M_{40} will be 10
and in the other case it will be 6.0 (which is which?). Field of
vision would be significantly greater with the eye nearer the lens.

References

Bennett, A.G. and Rabbetts, R.B. (1989) *Clinical Visual Optics*, Butterworths,
London, pp. 42 and 300

Farrall, H. (1991) *Optometric Management of Visual Handicap*, Blackwell
Scientific, Oxford, pp. 77, 83 and 87

Sloan, L.L. (1977) *Reading Aids for the Partially Sighted*, Williams and Wilkins,
Baltimore, pp. 20–22 and 27

Sloan, L.L. and Habel, A. (1956) Reading aids for the partially blind. *Am J
Ophthalmol*, **42**, 863–872

4 A young man is corrected for distance vision by spectacles which have the Rx +3.00 DS/–4.00 DC × 180. He may prefer a different astigmatic correction when reading at 33 cm. Which one of the following alternatives is most likely to be true?

   A Any difference would probably be greater if cycloplegia and an extra +3.00 DS for reading were to be used

   B Less than –4.00 DC will probably be preferred at 33 cm

   C More than –4.00 DC will probably be preferred at 33 cm

   D Any difference (an increase or a decrease in cylinder power) would probably have been greater had the distance Rx been –10.00 DS/–4.00 DC × 180

5 Tests of bichromatic or duochrome types for spherical refractive errors are covered by British Standard BS 3668 (1963). Which of the following suggestions is the correct one?

   A Two filters are used in conjunction with standard illuminant A (tungsten) and they should have weighted peaks of transmittance at approximately: (i) $555 - 75 = 480$ nm; and (ii) $555 + 75 = 630$ nm

   B An eye under cycloplegia sees the red part of the display clearly through +1.00 DS. A lens of +0.50 DS would be more likely than –0.50 DS to bring the green part into sharp focus

   C A protanope is likely to say that the green and red parts of the test are equally bright when they are equally in focus

   D Referring to an equal energy spectrum seen by a standard observer, his relative luminous efficiency curve must be modified by the energy distribution of the spectrum of tungsten light used on the test, in order that the maximum moves from 555 to 570 nm

4 Item C is the most likely, on account of the use of accommodation and of spectacles at a significant vertex distance. This is related to the 'accommodative demands' by each of the principal meridians being different, just as a (spectacle) corrected myope tends to need less accommodation than a (spectacle) corrected hyperope. There is a useful approximation by W. Swaine in which

$$\frac{\text{Near vision cyl.}}{\text{Distance vision cyl.}} = \left[\frac{1 + dA}{1 - dS} \right]^2$$

where d is vertex distance in m, A is assumed accommodation in use and S is distance spherical correction. Hence the $-10.00\,\text{DS}$ would incline to induce a greater difference than the $+3.00\,\text{DS}$.

References

Allen, R.J. *et al.* (1991) *Eye Examination and Refraction*, Blackwell Scientific, Oxford, pp. 112–114

Amos, J.F. (1991) *Clinical Procedures in Optometry* (ed. J.B. Eskridge), Lippincott, Philadelphia, p. 195

Bennett, A.G. and Rabbetts, R.B. (1989) *Clinical Visual Optics*, Butterworths, London, p. 150

Fletcher, R.J. (1952) Astigmatic accommodation. *Br J Physiol Opt*, **9**, 8–32

5 In fact, in A, peaks of 535 nm and 620 nm are what is required. Bennett (1963, p. 293) and Bennett and Rabbetts (1989, p. 347) point out the following: ocular chromatic aberration places 535 nm approximately $+0.25\,\text{D}$ from 570 nm and 620 nm about $-0.25\,\text{D}$ from 570 nm. These are 35 and 50 nm from the 'zero' dioptric position.

Item B is the minus lens which would be the better choice, even if not exact. As to item C, a protanope should have lowered sensitivity to the red light; see Bennett (1963, p. 295), and Fletcher and Voke (1985, p. 168).

The correct choice is D, on account of the red bias of tungsten light; see Bennett (1963, p. 293) and Fletcher and Voke (1985, p. 264).

References

Bennett, A.G. (1963) The theory of bichromatic tests. *Optician*, **146**, 293 and 295

Bennett, A.G. and Rabbetts, R.B. (1989) *Clinical Visual Optics*, 2nd edn, Butterworths, London

Fletcher, R. and Voke, J. (1985) *Defective Colour Vision*, Hilger, Bristol, pp. 168 and 264

Still, D.C. (1991) *Eye Examination and Refraction* (eds R.J. Allen *et al.*), Blackwell Scientific, Oxford, pp. 179–180

6 Presbyopia correction is an important feature of optometric practice and one of the items listed below is correct, while the others are incorrect

    A The elasticity of the lens nucleus and of the cortex rapidly decrease and the elasticity of the capsule increases as age progresses

    B An eye with a (spectacle plane) amplitude of accommodation of 3.00 D views an object 40 cm from a spectacle lens of +4.00 D, which incorporates a +1.00 add. The object is seen clearly, thus one half of the amplitude of accommodation should be in operation

    C The zonule (of Zinn) is not elastic and does not act as an antagonist to the ciliary muscle

    D The ciliary muscle does not change significantly with age

7 The effective power of a spectacle lens, referred to the corneal plane is influenced by the vertex distance and the back vertex power (BVP) of the lens. There is a certain power, combined with (say) a typical vertex distance of 14 mm, above which the effective power and the BVP are significantly different. Assuming a vertex distance of 14 mm and a difference of 0.25 D to be significant, for which of the following BV powers would that difference be present in the effective power at the cornea?

    A +2.00 D
    B +3.00 D
    C +4.00 D
    D +5.00 D

8 A useful stereoscope for diagnosis and orthoptics consists of two 9 prism dioptre (pd) prisms, base out. A pair of stereograms is used in the form of two vertical lines, 60 cm apart, seen by a person with a PD of 60 mm through the prisms. The prisms are 37 mm from the centres of rotation of the eyes. The line objects are 333 mm from the (thin) prisms. How much convergence is needed to fuse the images of the two lines?

    A 16.2 pd
    B 18 pd
    C 37 pd (since for near vision a prism has an increased effective power)
    D 8.1 pd (since for near vision a prism has a reduced effective power)

6 One half of the spectacle accommodation, exercised in the spectacle plane, would be 1.50 D. The distance spectacle correction is clearly +3.00 D, the vergence leaving the lens during distance vision. The vergence leaving the +4.00 D lens during near vision is only +1.50 D but the 1.50 D of spectacle accommodation compensates for the missing vergence. Thus item B should be chosen. Stafford (1994) and Stark (1987) indicate how the other items are incorrect. Bennett and Rabbetts (1989) show a related approach to the calculation.

References

Bennett, A.G. and Rabbetts, R.B. (1989) *Clinical Visual Optics*, 2nd edn, Butterworths, London, pp. 142–143

Stafford, A. (1994) *Optician*, **208**, 25

Stark, L. (1987) In *Presbyopia* (eds L. Stark and G. Obrecht), Professional Press (Fairchild), New York, pp. 274–278

7 The +4.00 D BVP has an effective power at the cornea of +4.25 D, so C should be chosen, although the +3.00 D BVP has an effective power of +3.12 D. All powers are given correct to 0.12 D.

Refer to any text on visual optics or most contact lens texts or Borish (1970). Note that, working in mm, 1000/4 = 250 mm, then 250 − 14 = 236 mm, when 1000/236 = 4.24 or 4.25 corrected.

Reference

Borish, I.M. (1970) *Clinical Refraction*, 3rd edn, Professional Press, Chicago, p. 1063

8 Since each prism deviates light by 9 pd, but (under the circumstances) has an effective power less than this amount at the centre of rotation of the eye, each eye has to rotate nasally by 8.1 pd. Item A is the convergence needed, the sum of the movements of the two eyes. Note that the effective power is not the same for distant and near objects.

References

Bennett, A.G. (1968) *Ophthalmic Lenses*. Hatton Press, London, pp. 207–208

Bennett, A.G. and Rabbetts, R.B. (1989) *Clinical Visual Optics*, 2nd edn, Butterworths, London, p. 286 (noting that the effective prism power is 5–10% less in near vision; see also p. 327)

Brooks, C.W. and Riley, H.D. (1994) Effect of prescribed prism on monocular interpupillary distances and fitting heights for progressive add lenses. *Optom and Vision Science*, **71**, 401–407 (note pp. 404–405)

9 A Maddox rod (or 'groove') is used in front of the right eye while the subject views a spot light with the left eye. A 5 pd plano prism is used to measure the vertical phoria (with the streak image seen horizontal) and the horizontal phoria when the streak appears vertical. In each case, the prism is held exactly along 127 degrees, standard notation, with its base 'up and out'. What are the appropriate phorias, as measured?

A   3 pd R hyper with 6 pd exo
B   6 pd R hyper with 3 pd eso
C   3 pd L hyper with 4 pd eso
D   3 pd R hyper with 3 pd eso

10 Despite the (limited) advantages of 'phoropter' or 'refracting unit' devices, trial case lenses remain an important part of optometric equipment. A 1956 committee made recommendations which influenced British Standard 3162 (1969) which dealt with trial case lenses. Which of the following is most correct?

A   Plus spheres must be biconvex and placed in the rear cell of the trial frame
B   Cylinder lenses should be in the rear cell
C   Plus spheres must be planoconvex, placed with the convex surface nearer to the eye
D   Relatively high plus trial lenses have the same optical effect when used for distant or near objects

11 Visual acuity variation using different retinal locations is important in several clinical situations, such as 'eccentric fixation'. Opinions have differed as to the expected variations, particularly in normal eyes, but it is usually possible to fix reasonable limits. Which of the following is most likely to represent the range of visual acuity for a retinal location 5 degrees nasally away from the fovea?

A   Between 6/36 and 6/60
B   Between 6/60 and 3/36
C   Between 6/6 and 6/9 but probably nearer 6/9
D   Between 6/18 and 6/36 but probably nearer 6/18

Visual optics: Answers

9 By graphical construction, starting with a 5 cm line along 127 degrees and measuring 4 cm and 3 cm along the horizontal and vertical ordinates, the prism can be found to be a compound of vertical and horizontal prisms, showing item C to be correct.

References

Bennett, A.G. (1968) *Ophthalmic Lenses*, Hatton Press, London, pp. 109–111
Jalie, M. and Wray, I. (1979) *Practical Ophthalmic Lenses*, Butterworths, London, pp. 110–111

10 Item C is most correct, with each of the other items on insecure ground when compared with the Standard's requirements. However, it is usually possible to measure the BVP of any combination of trial case lenses, provided that the data are correctly applied!

References

Bennett, A.G. (1968) *Ophthalmic Lenses*, Hatton Press, London, pp. 177–179
British Scientific Instrument Research Association (1949) The back vertex power of trial lens combinations. *Optician*, **118**, 452–455
Fletcher, R. (1991) In *Eye Examination and Refraction* (eds R.J. Allen *et al.*), Blackwell Scientific, Oxford, pp. 69–70

11 In Ciuffreda *et al.* (1991) the difficulties of the answer are elaborated but item D is probably a reasonable choice. Note how many orthoptics texts avoid the issue!

References

Bennett, A.G. and Rabbetts, R.B. (1989) *Clinical Visual Optics*, 2nd edn, Butterworths, London, p. 43
Ciuffreda, K.J. *et al.* (1991) *Amblyopia, Basic and Clinical Aspects*, Butterworth-Heinemann, Boston, pp. 343–348

12 A keratoprosthesis has been designed, to be made as a 7.7 mm
long cylinder to be inserted into the cornea into an aphakic eye.
The radius of the front surface is to be 7.54 mm and the distance
from the back surface of the plastics material (refractive index
(*n*) 1.490) is to be 21.75 mm from the retina. The vitreous cavity
has a refractive index 1.336. The 'principal planes' should be
placed in the optimum position to achieve the maximum field of
view for the patient, who is unsuitable for a corneal graft.

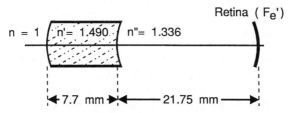

Fig. 1.3 Arrangement of corneal prosthesis relative to the retina
which is at F_e'.

Which of the following is the most likely radius for the back
surface of the cylinder, nearer to the retina as indicated in Figure
1.3? Assume that distant objects are to be seen.

A   7.7 mm
B   8.95 mm
C   4.23 mm
D   22.22 mm

13 A model eye is made of glass, refractive index 1.50, in the form
of a sphere with a radius of 10 mm. To imitate an eye and to use
it for retinoscopy practice, the sphere is completely painted
orange, the orange paint is covered with black paint, but no
paint is applied to a 4 mm diameter 'pupil' at one place.
Retinoscopy (at 1 m distance) is now carried out with a plane
mirror instrument along the optical axis of the 'eye'. What is the
power of the thin lens which must be in contact with the centre
of the 'pupil' in order to give reversal of the reflex movement?

A   −50 DS
B   −25 DS
C   +30 DS
D   +26 DS

12 Item C is most suitable since the vergence reaching the back surface of the prosthesis is +97.9 D. The back vertex focal length of the prosthesis is to be 21.75 mm. The power of the back surface (using the difference between the two refractive indices) should be −36.6 D, approximately.

References

Barron, B.A. (1988) In *The Cornea* (eds H.E. Kaufman *et al.*), Churchill Livingstone, New York, pp. 787–803

Waltman, S.R. *et al.* (1988) *Surgery of the Eye*, Churchill Livingstone, New York, pp. 299–306

Wright, K.W. and Ryan, S.J. (1992) *Corneal and Refractive Surgery*, Lippincott, Philadelphia, pp. 107–124

13 As the ocular power is +50 D, the eye would have to be 1500/50 mm (30 mm) long to be emmetropic, but the axial length is only 20 mm, which corresponds to a required vergence of +75 D. So the eye is 25 D hyperopic. Add to this a 'working distance' lens of +1.00 D and the thin lens power of +26 D is obtained, as in item D.

Reference

See virtually any standard visual optics text, including those indicated elsewhere in this book.

14 The effect on retinal image sizes of the positions (vertex distances) of spectacle corrections for anisometropia may follow Knapp's law, according to the state of the axial lengths of a patient's eyes. Suppose that a patient with spectacle corrections R −1.00 DS and L −8.00 DS is reasonably happy with his binocular vision. He then has either a contact lens correction for both eyes or refractive surgery to reduce his left prescription to −1.00 DS, combined with a contact lens for his RE. Then he complains of seeing objects significantly larger with one eye. Suggest the most likely explanation from among the following.

A   The retinal images are made more equal in size, but stretching of the perifoveal retina which previously existed in his more myopic eye reduced the number of receptors per square millimetre

B   The left eye myopia is not likely to have been caused by axial length

C   The patient is complaining without any possible cause

D   Knapp's law was based on unsound theoretical understanding of visual optics

15 An emmetropic partially sighted child uses a monocular telescope for viewing distant objects. The telescope is made from a +20.00 DS lens and a −40.00 DS lens, separated by 25 mm but the focus cannot be changed. The minus lens is held 15 mm from the cornea and the child looks through the telescope at an object 40 cm from the front lens. Treat both lenses as 'thin' and identify from among the choices below how much accommodation (referred to the corneal plane) must be used for this near vision task.

A   Between 7.00 and 8.00 D

B   Between 20.00 and 22.00 D

C   Between 2.00 and 4.00 D

D   Between 10.00 and 12.00 D

14 Probably the first term can be taken most seriously, particularly if ophthalmoscopic signs over some years support unilateral axial myopia. The approach (see Grosvenor and Flom, 1991) would suppose adaptation to (axial) optical magnification offset by 'neural minification' from retinal stretching; this might or might not be upset by relocation of the optical correction.

Note the uncertainty of predicting the outcome of such a corneal plane correction but the greater ease of experimenting with a contact lens rather than surgery!

References

Applegate, R.A. and Howland, H.C. (1993) Magnification and visual acuity in refractive surgery. *Arch Ophthalmol*, **111**, 1335–1342

Bennett, A.G. and Rabbetts, R.B. (1989) *Clinical Visual Optics*, Butterworths, London, pp. 284 and 313

Grosvenor, T. and Flom, M.C. (1991) *Refractive Anomalies*, Butterworth-Heinemann, Boston, pp. 190–194

Winn, B. *et al.* (1988) Reduced aniseikonia in axial anisometropia with contact lens correction. *Ophthal Physiol Opt*, **8**, 341–344

15 The telescope places what might at first be considered extravagant demands on accommodation, but not over 8 D. Hence item A is a suitable choice. The reasoning might be that light reaches the +20.00 DS diverging –2.50 D. Thus, light leaves the +20.00 DS converging +17.5 D and reaches the –40.00 DS converging +31.11 D, so leaves the –40.00 DS diverging –8.89 D, thus reaching the cornea diverging –7.84 D.

Light from a distant object would have reached the cornea with zero vergence so the corneal plane accommodation needed is 7.84 D.

Reference

Obstfeld, H. (1982) *Optics in Vision*, 2nd edn, Butterworth Scientific, London, pp. 183–186

16 Following cataract surgery an optometrist may be involved with the refractive state of the eye at different stages. Which of the following items is the most correct one?

  A   It usually takes about 15 months before a satisfactory and stable spectacle correction can be prescribed after a cataract operation

  B   Following a phakoemulsification procedure there is invariably some astigmatism and when corrected by a plus cylinder the axis of this cylinder is usually at 45 degrees away from any tight corneal suture

  C   If compression from tight suturing is noted, perhaps by a photokeratoscope, with excessive 'with the rule' astigmatism, an opposite error in the astigmatic state is best avoided by very early removal of any tight suture

  D   Postoperatively, the principal meridians of the cornea may not be at 90 degrees to each other. Therefore a 'one-position' type keratometer should be used in two 'positions' to assess the corneal refractive contribution

17 While every eye must be regarded as an individual, subjected to various influences, there are well known trends which change the refractive state of the eye as age progresses. Leaving aside presbyopia, to which decade of life is Figure 1.4 most likely to refer, assuming a 'mean spherical spectacle correction', in Europeans, to be involved?

  A   5–15 years
  B   10–20 years
  C   30–40 years
  D   45–55 years

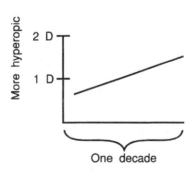

Fig. 1.4 Typical refractive changes over a decade.

16 Really the only correct item is D.

References

Davey, K. (1993) Refraction after cataract surgery. *Br J Optom Disp*, **1**, 135–136
Douthwaite, W.A. and Hurst, M.A. (1993) *Cataract detection, measurement and management in optometric practice*. Butterworth-Heinemann, Oxford, p. 101
Troutman, R.C. and Swinger, C.A. (1988) In *Surgery of the Eye* (eds S.R. Waltman *et al.*), Churchill Livingstone, New York, p. 295

17 Since the change is a gradual one towards about one dioptre more hyperopia, or less myopia, item D is most likely. The trend might have been considered to refer to the period up to about 5 years, but this was not an option; the 'down slope' to myopia tends to come at two other periods of life.

References

Allen, R.J., Fletcher, R. and Still, D.C. (1991) *Eye Examination and Refraction*, Blackwell Scientific, Oxford, pp. 116–121
Bennett, A.G. and Rabbetts, R.B. (1989) *Clinical Visual Optics*, Butterworths, London, p. 494
Grosvenor, T. and Flom, M.C. (1991) *Refractive Anomalies*, Butterworth-Heinemann, Boston, pp. 142–144
Sorsby, A. *et al.* (1961) Refraction and its components during the growth of the eye from the age of three. *Spec Report Med Res Council* 301, HMSO, London

18 Iseikonic or 'size' lenses have some role in assisting certain binocular problems and the principles often apply to less unusual cases. Select from the following items the one most likely to be a correct guide in spectacle prescribing.

A   A lens (centre thickness 4 mm) has surface powers of +8 DS and −6 DS. Its spectacle magnification effect will decrease by just over 1% if its thickness is increased to 7 mm.

B   Assuming that the effective power at the eye is kept constant by a slight variation of the front surface power, the increase in thickness of the lens mentioned above would *increase* (and not decrease) the magnification by about 1.2%

C   An increase in the back surface power of a lens (maintaining BVP) tends to have the opposite effect to that produced by an increase in thickness

D   An increase in vertex distance (correcting BVP) decreases the spectacle magnification of a high plus lens

19 An observer holds a series of Scheiner discs in front of one eye, occluding the other eye. The discs are in the front focal plane of the eye. The apertures are all 1 mm in diameter but on different discs they have different separations, always along 180 degrees. He observes the sky, seeing one of the three appearances illustrated in Figure 1.5 through each of three different discs. Which of the following suggestions is the correct one?

A   The separation of the centres of the apertures equals the pupil diameter when he sees (ii)

B   He is myopic more than $1000/f_e$ in mm, in dioptres

C   If the observer uncovers his other eye he should describe a change from (ii) to (iii)

D   The separation of the apertures when he sees (ii) equals his pupil radius

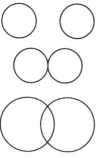

Fig. 1.5 Alternative subjective appearances of blur circles.

18 All the suggestions except B express the opposite of the accepted effects. With this proviso, all could be considered in the context of manipulating retinal image size. Item B is given in the correct form and should be chosen.

References

Adams, T. (1968) The correction of aniseikonia: two case records. *Optician*, **156**, 417–418 (A practical issue, simply described)

Allen, R.J., Fletcher, R. and Still, D.C. (1991) *Eye Examination and Refraction*, Blackwell Scientific, Oxford, p. 130

Bennett, A.G. (1937) The fundamentals of iseikonic lenses. *Optician*: various pages in January and February, forming a classical account of great value

Brown, R.M. and Enoch, J.M. (1970) Combined rules of thumb in aniseikonic prescription. *Am J Ophthalmol*, **43**, 118–126

Cholerton, M. (1948) *Some Aspects of Oculo-refractive Technique*, Hammond, London, p. 46

19 Item B is absurd, while C suggests that his pupils would become larger and not smaller, on account of 'light reflexes'. Item A is the logically correct one, rather than D.

References

Bennett, A.G. and Rabbetts, R.B. (1989) *Clinical Visual Optics*, 2nd edn, Butterworths, London, pp. 84–85

Lowenfeld, I.E. (1993) *The Pupil*, Vol. I, Iowa State UP, Ames, p. 26 (*note* this massive text is remarkably informative)

Obstfeld, H. (1982) *Optics in Vision*, 2nd edn, Butterworths, London, pp. 92–93

Rubin, M.L. and Walls, G.L. (1965) *Studies in Physiological Optics*, Thomas, Springfield, pp. 70–71

20 A person looks at a point which is 150 mm below the level of the 'primary position' of the line of sight in a vertical plane 400 mm from the spectacle plane, the latter being 26 mm from the centre of rotation of the right eye and 25 mm from the centre of rotation of the left eye. The distance PD is 65 mm. The spectacle lenses are R −10.00 DS and L −6.00 DS, with the optical centres placed for distance vision. With respect to the 'near visual points' under these circumstances (the position on each lens through which an eye sees the point object), which of the following is most likely to be correct?

A The near visual point on the right lens will be higher than that on the left lens

B The near visual point on the left lens will be higher than that on the right lens

C The near visual points on each lens will be at exactly the same distance below the optical centres

D The near visual point on the left lens will be more than 13 mm below the optical centre

21 Neutral filters are widely used in optometric investigation, for example with amblyopia, there being a conventional method of grading the density of such filters. Which of the following is most likely to be correct?

A Neutral density (ND) = $\log_{10} 1/\text{transmission}$

B Assuming that a 0.60 ND filter transmits nearly 25% of incident light, a 0.30 ND filter will transmit about 12.5%

C If a 0.20 ND filter is placed in contact with a 1.00 ND filter, the transmission through both is very nearly the same as that through a filter of ND 0.50

D A single polarizing filter, rotated around the visual axis, will provide an ND filter of variable transmission, regardless of the characteristics of a source of light which is viewed

Visual optics: Answers

20 Simple calculations and/or a scale diagram should indicate that the virtual image at which each eye looks is nearer and smaller for the more myopic eye, the eye which looks through a near visual point nearer to the distance optical centre, or higher. This suggests that item A is correct, while B and C are incorrect. The figure suggested in D is excessive.

References
Bennett, A.G. (1968) *Ophthalmic Lenses*, Hatton Press, London, p. 210
Bennett, A.G. and Rabbetts, R.B. (1989) *Clinical Visual Optics*, 2nd edn, Butterworths, London, pp. 290–291
Borish, I.M. (1954) *Clinical Refraction*, 3rd edn, Professional Press, Chicago, pp. 424–428 (No account is taken of the spectacle lens power!)
Obstfeld, H. (1982) *Optics in Vision*, 2nd edn, Butterworth Scientific, London, pp. 282–291

21 Item A, alone, is correct. In B, 0.60 ND transmits about 25% but 0.30 ND transmits about 50%. Adding 0.20 ND to 1.00 ND produces 1.20 ND, transmitting about 6.30%, while ND 0.50 transmits 31.6%. As for D, few polarizing filters are very neutral when crossed with another, but also two such filters rotated against each other are needed to vary the total transmission.

References
Cline, D. *et al.* (1989) *Dictionary of Visual Science*, Chilton, Radnor, Pennsylvania, p. 179
Crawford, B.H. *et al.* (eds) (1968) *Techniques of Photostimulation in Biology*, North-Holland, Amsterdam, pp. 89–90
Le Grand, Y. (1968) *Light, Colour and Vision*, 2nd edn, Chapman & Hall, London, pp. 38 and 195

22 There is a well recognized term (often used incorrectly) relating to an individual spherical spectacle lens. It refers to the power of a surface (either, as appropriate) which has been selected in order to determine the 'form' of that lens. The term also applies to a surface power which is common to all the lenses in a range of lenses of different powers. Select the term from the following.

A Nominal base curve
B Principal power(s)
C Meniscus
D Base curve

22 The term is named in item D, as *base curve*; this is 06-003 in BS 3521: Part 1 (1991).

Reference

BS 3521: Part 1 (1991) British Standards Institution, Milton Keynes, p. 18

23   A good spectacle prescription stands or falls by good dispensing, both controlling several aspects of the visual optics of the situation. Figure 1.6 shows two lenses 'boxed' for measurement, with the bridge region of a frame indicated. The extent to which the lenses rest in the groove of the rim is suggested.

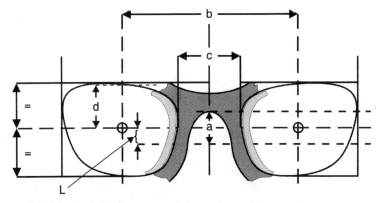

Fig. 1.6 Two fitted lenses with box dimensions and part of frame. The lighter part of the shading represents the part of the bridge which, being grooved, covers the lenses.

Five dimensions are shown: a, b, c, d and L; one is not given a standard letter. Which one of the following suggestions is correct, according to British Standards?

A   The centre line of each lens is shown as b. The vertical lens size of each lens is shown as d. The crest height of the frame is shown as a

B   The centre line of each lens is shown by b. The bridge width is shown by c. The boxed lens size of each lens is shown by d

C   The bridge height (from the bridge width line) is shown by a. The dimension L, from the bridge width line to the horizontal centre line, equals 5 mm. The distance between lenses (DBL) = c

D   The centre line of the frame is shown as b. The bridge width is measured along the line between the lens centres. The bridge height is shown as L

23 It is only the three statements given in item C which are correct. All others are false. *Note*: among the North American terms in use, the British Standard DBL is sometimes called 'bridge size'!

References
Brooks, C.W. (1992) *Understanding Lens Surfacing*, Butterworth-Heinemann, Oxford
BS 3521: Part 2 (1991) British Standards Institution, Milton Keynes

24 There are recognized tolerances for the optical properties of mounted spectacle lenses, for which an optometrist bears some responsibility. Which of the following sets of tolerances is the only correct one?

    A   For non-progressive power lenses, with 'highest absolute lens powers' of between 3.25 D and 4.00 D sphere, and a cylindrical correction of 4.00 D or less, the permitted tolerance is ±0.12 D

    B   For non-progressive lenses with a highest absolute power of between 3.25 D and 4.00 D in either principal meridian, the tolerance is ±0.25 D for cylindrical corrections greater than 0.75 DC and ±0.18 D for corrections up to 0.75 DC

    C   For progressive power lenses with highest absolute power of 6.50 DS for each meridian combined with a cylindrical power of up to 4.00 D, the tolerance is ±0.25 D

    D   For progressive power lenses with highest absolute power up to 3.00 DS for each meridian combined with an associated cylindrical power of up to 0.75 D, the tolerance is ±0.18 D

25 While patients sometimes manage tolerably well with incorrect spectacle corrections, this is not ideal. Therefore there are British Standard tolerances for the cylinder axes of mounted spectacles. The following suggestions refer only to the cylinder axes of non-progressive power lenses. Which one is the correct item?

    A   For a cylinder of power 1.00 DC the tolerance is ±1.5 degrees

    B   For a cylinder of power 2.00 DC the tolerance is ±2 degrees

    C   For a cylinder of power 2.00 DC the tolerance is ±5 degrees

    D   For a cylinder of power 2.00 DC the tolerance is ±1.5 degrees

Visual optics: Answers

24 According to BS 2738 (1989) it is only item A which is correct. All the other suggestions are at variance with the Standard.

Reference

BS 2738: Part 1 (1989) British Standards Institution, Milton Keynes, p. 3

25 Item D is the only correct one, according to BS 2728 (1989)

Reference

BS 2728: Part 1 (1989) British Standards Institution, Milton Keynes, p. 4

26 Round spectacle lenses mounted in frames have been known sometimes to rotate; when they are astigmatic lenses the results can be disturbing. There is a standard manner of permanent marking of round lenses by which unwanted rotation can be detected. Which of the following possibilities is the correct one?

A   Two marks are made, next to the joint, symmetrically one on either side of the joint line on the right lens and one mark is made on the joint line of the left lens

B   One mark is made on the joint line on the back surface of each thermally toughened lens; the fact that the lenses are unlikely to be transposed making one mark on each sufficient

C   On the right lens one mark is made on the back surface at the joint line, two such marks being made symmetrically on either side of the joint line on the back surface of the left lens

D   On the right lens one mark is made on the back surface at 6 o'clock, two marks being made, similarly placed, on the back of the left lens

27 The optical centres of a pair of spectacle lenses, for distance vision, are mounted in a plastics frame so that they are 63 mm apart on a horizontal line, after a certain amount of prescribed prism has been neutralized. Which of the following terms is the correct one for this distance of 63 mm?

A   Optical PD
B   Optical centres (OCs)
C   Optical centre distance (OCD)
D   Standard optical centre position

28 Which of the following is the correct interpretation of the British Standard and International (ISO) term *boxed centre* of a lens?

A   The point of location of the optical centre in the absence of any prescribed prism or after such prism has been neutralized

B   The assumed position of the visual point on a lens, when distance vision is in use and the eyes are in the primary position

C   The midpoint of the rectangle containing the lens shape

26 Item C is correct, according to BS 2738: Part 1: (1989). Note that thermally toughened lenses are weakened by being scratched.

Reference
BS 2738: Part 1 (1989) British Standards Institution, Milton Keynes, p. 7

27 Item C is correct since according to BS 3521: Part 1: (1991) both A and B are 'deprecated' terms. Item D is rather the term for a reference point specific to one lens of a certain shape.

Reference
BS 3521: Part 1 (1991) British Standards Institution, Milton Keynes

28 According to BS 3521: Part 1: (1991), BS 3199 (1992) and ISO 8624 (1991), item A, in a reworded form, refers to *centration point* and item B similarly refers to *distance visual point*. Item C is the correct one which refers to *boxed centre* in the 1991 BS.

References
BS 3521: Part 1: (1991) British Standards Institution, Milton Keynes
BS 3199 (1992) British Standards Institution, Milton Keynes
ISO 8624 (1991) International Standards Organization

29 In some lenses the vertical extent of a bifocal segment nowhere extends to the lens periphery. This dimension can be measured (as appropriate) through the top or bottom of the segment, as shown with the letter V in Figure 1.7(i). Which term is used correctly to describe the vertical extent of a D segment bifocal which does not extend to the periphery?

A Segment height
B Segment depth
C Segment top position
D Segment drop

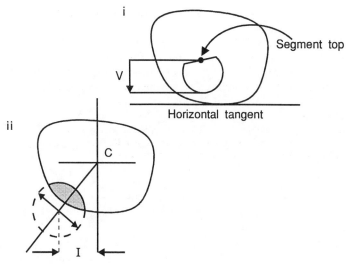

Fig. 1.7 Features of bifocal lenses: (i) straight top; (ii) inset.

30 In Figure 1.7(ii) the distance indicated by the letter I is shown as the horizontal distance between two vertical lines. One of these lines extends downwards from the distance centration point; the other extends downwards from the midpoint of the diameter of a bifocal segment. What is the correct term for distance I?

A Geometrical inset
B Inset
C Optical inset
D Conventional inset

29 Item A is correct. The other terms refer to other dimensions, as described in BS 3521: Part 1: (1991).

Reference
BS 3521: Part 1: (1991) British Standards Institution, Milton Keynes

30 A is the correct term. All the other terms can also be found in BS 3521: Part 1: (1991) relating to other features.

Reference
BS 3521: Part 1: (1991) British Standards Institution, Milton Keynes

31 A focimeter, normally used to measure powers of spectacle
lenses, can be used to determine the 'addition power' of a 'front
surface' bifocal. Vertex powers of both the major area and the
segment area of the lens are used. Figure 1.8 suggests different
ways in which vertex powers could be measured, with a view to
determining the 'addition power'. Which is correct?

A   Front vertex power (FVP) of segment area minus back
vertex power (BVP) of major area
B   BVP of segment area minus BVP of main area
C   FVP of segment area minus FVP of main area
D   BVP of segment area minus FVP of main area

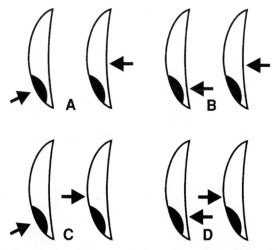

Fig. 1.8 Standard and non-standard measurements of bifocal
segment. The lens shown twice as A has its addition measured using
the front vertex power of the segment and the back vertex power of
the distance Rx. The lens at B is measured using both back vertex
powers. Lens C involves two front vertex power measurements. Lens
D has the segment back vertex power and the distance front vertex
power compared.

Visual optics: Answers

31 Item C, which involves two front vertex powers, is correct. The other possibilities are incorrect, according to BS 2738: Part 1: (1989).

Reference

BS 2738: Part 1: (1989) British Standards Institution, Milton Keynes

32 The size of a retinal lesion is likely to correspond to the extent of a visual field defect. Which of the following possibilities, correct to the nearest 0.5 mm, is most likely to be the size of the (sharp) retinal image in this situation? The eye is a myopic 'reduced' eye, unaccommodating and with a refractive index of 4/3, having a radius of curvature of 5 mm. It observes an object 2 mm in size which is situated at its far point, this being 75 mm from the eye.

A   2.50 mm
B   1.50 mm
C   0.50 mm
D   2.00 mm

33 In 1954 an Australian clinician J. Lederer described a series of glass spectacle lenses with a diameter of less than 40 mm and a thickness up to 9 mm, which were useful for visually handicapped patients. The influence of the designs is present today. Which of the following combinations of surface powers did he design to provide a nominal magnification of 5 times?

A   +17.50 and +3.00 D
B   +20.00 and +16.00 D
C   +14.75 and −3.00 D
D   +25.00 and −10.00 D

Visual optics: Answers

32 The correct item is C, the size being 0.50 mm. Figure 1.9 shows similar triangles and a familiar formula, m = K/K′, might be used to find that m = 1/4, having found the axial length of the eye. The following steps are useful:

(i) Find power of eye (using r and *n′*) as +66.66 D.
(ii) Far point at 75 mm is −13.33 D near, which equals ocular refraction K.
(iii) The calculations above give K′, the dioptric length of the eye as +53.32 D, whence K/K′ = 1/4 (minus in this case), or length of eye = k′ = *n′*/K′ = 25 mm.
(iv) So C in the Figure is 20 mm from retina and 80 mm from object.
(v) Similar triangles give image 1/4 size of object.

Alternatively, since object subtends 2.50 prism dioptres at C, so does the sharp image and at 20 mm from C this would be

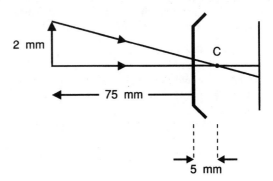

Fig. 1.9 Reduced eye with retinal image size.

0.50 mm.

33 Item A is correct, not the others. Application of the relatively simplistic F/4 relationship, sometimes a reasonable starting point, should give the correct clue.

References

Bier, N. (1960) *Correction of Subnormal Vision*, Butterworths, London, pp. 65–69
Lederer, J. (1954) The Lederer lenses – a new development in subnormal vision aids. *Aust J Optom*, **37**, 297
Lederer, J. (1955) A new development in aids in subnormal vision. *Br J Physiol Opt*, **12**, 184

34 Which two of the following terms, while not being 'an integral part of the boxing system' described in ISO 8624: (1991) (E) are included in that Standard because they are important in the context?

A   Horizontal lens size
B   Bridge width
C   Distance between centres
D   Bridge height

35 Modern refractive surgical procedures require an understanding of the relative positions of the entrance pupil of the eye and the optical zone of the corneal surface. Thus the alignment of a photokeratoscope or videokeratographical apparatus with respect to the subject's fixation is critical. Which one of the following statements is accurate?

A   In the living eye the pupil is generally displaced temporally. This may cause the observer to align the axis of a videokeratoscope nearer to the line of sight
B   In the living eye the pupil is often displaced nasally, which may cause the observer to align the axis of a videokeratoscope nearer to the line of sight
C   In the living eye the pupil is often displaced nasally, which may tend to deflect the axis of a videokeratograph away from the line of sight
D   The pupillary axis (from the pupil centre and perpendicular to the cornea) coincides with the line of sight, ensuring that the videokeratograph axis lies along the visual axis

34 Items B and D should be chosen. Bridge width is the minimum distance between the pad surfaces of a frame, measured on the *bridge width line* which lies 5 mm below the horizontal centre line, the latter being taken through the two boxed centres. Bridge height, a vertical distance, goes from the bridge width line to the point of intersection with the lower edge of the bridge, along the vertical symmetry axis. Note that the 'bridge width' has replaced the older term 'distance between rims'.

35 Item B is accurate but since not all eyes have this feature it is usually the line of sight which is of critical interest in surgery as the important reference axis. The other items are inaccurate and misleading.

References

Bennett, A.G. and Rabbetts, R.B. (1989) *Clinical Visual Optics*, 2nd edn, Butterworths, London, pp. 264–266

Mandell, R.B. (1994) Apparent pupil displacement in videokeratography. *CLAO J*, **20**, 123–127

36 Accommodation by emmetropic subjects enables them to read at distances nearer than arm's length, until presbyopia becomes significant. Various estimates of how much of a person's amplitude of accommodation can be sustained with comfort include 2/3 of the amplitude. Assuming that Duane's (1922) data for accommodation at different ages are valid, a 30-year-old person is likely to have an amplitude between 6 and 11 dioptres; at 50 the range would be between 1 and 3 dioptres. Assuming that all the subjects have pupils about 4 mm in diameter and are reading under 300 lx., which of the following proposals is the most likely?

A Using 2/3 of the amplitude of accommodation, an emmetropic subject aged 45 is likely to be able to read small letters no nearer than 75 cm away from his eyes

B Using all his accommodation, an emmetropic subject aged 45 is likely to be able to read small letters no nearer than between 17 and 50 cm from his eyes, or (using a mean amplitude) about 25 cm away

C An emmetropic man aged 53 years is likely to have almost exactly one third of the amplitude of accommodation of an emmetrope aged 19 years

D Using all his amplitude of accommodation. an emmetrope aged 70 with an average amount of accommodation will probably be able to read small letters at 50 cm

E A 10-year-old emmetrope would normally have an amplitude of between 8 and 10 D of accommodation

37 Two types of ametropia have been differentiated by taking into account various factors; these include the relationships between axial length, corneal power, lens power and lens position. Which one of the following is most likely to be correct?

A 'Component' ametropia can lie between −4.00 D and +6.00 D. It is mainly the result of well correlated optical components of the eyes with such refractive errors

B In emmetropia, the mean value for axial length is more likely to be a little under 20 mm (with a standard deviation of 0.45) than a little over 24 mm (with a standard deviation of 0.85)

C Either hyperopia or myopia within the range +6.00 D to −4.00 D can often be caused by bad correlation between the optical components of an eye

D In animals, axial hyperopia has been experimentally found to be related to lack of a good retinal image caused by corneal scars or ptosis

36 Item B is the most likely. There are some remarkable exceptions and various influences can affect amplitude of accommodation and depth of field considerably.

References

Bennett, A.G. (1972) Variation of accommodation with age: a new graph. *Optician*, **12**, 197–198

Bennett, A.G. and Rabbetts, R.B. (1989) *Clinical Visual Optics*, 2nd edn, Butterworths, London, pp. 140–142

Wagstaff, D.F. (1966) The objective measurement of the amplitude of accommodation. *Optician*, **151**, 105–109

Weale, R.A. (1963) *The Aging Eye*, Lewis, London, p. 115

37 Item C should be chosen. In item B the smaller value refers to a fairly typical group of hyperopes, while it is the larger figure (over 24 mm) which was found for a group of over 100 emmetropes.

References

Bennett, A.G. and Rabbetts, R.B. (1989) *Clinical Visual Optics*, 2nd edn, Butterworths, London, pp. 489–495

Sorsby, A., Leary, G.A. and Richards, M.J. (1962) Correlation ametropia and component ametropia. *Vision Res*, **2**, 309–313

Stone, R.A. *et al.* (1990) In *Ciba Symposium ISS: Myopia and the Control of Eye Growth*, Wiley, Chichester, p.46

38 The axial length of a living eye can be determined with reasonable accuracy at different times in a person's life. Which one of the following suggestions is most likely to be correct, or do you suppose two to be very likely to be correct?

    A   An increase of 2.50 mm in axial length of a person's eye was found to decrease its hypermetropia by 3.50 D, leaving the spectacle correction at +0.50 D

    B   Elongation of an eye over several years of a myopic subject's life cannot be compensated by other optical features, such as corneal and lens powers

    C   The process known as 'emmetropization' is proven by the fact that a proportion of children develop myopia while others remain as hypermetropes

    D   It is the crystalline lens which is the least effective ocular component to be active in offsetting elongation of the axial length of an eye

39 A keratometer is calibrated for a refractive index of 1.3375. When used to measure the principal meridians of a certain cornea which has 'against-the-rule' toricity, it indicates the need for a correcting cylindrical lens of −4.00 DC axis 90. Which of the following pairs of meridional measurements would be most likely to be involved?

    A   7.94 mm along 90, with 8.65 mm along 180

    B   7.50 mm along 90, with 8.70 mm along 180

    C   7.50 mm along 180, with 8.23 mm along 90

    D   7.30 mm along 180, with 7.70 mm along 90

40 Refractive surgery of the cornea, such as radial keratotomy (RK) is carried out by several different procedures. The form of the cornea is altered to modify a refractive error. Which one of the following is most likely to be correct?

    A   Following RK there is a significant diurnal change in corneal curvature, which is usually a change of radius of approximately 0.40 mm

    B   RK tends to produce disability glare and this is suffered mostly by subjects with relatively large pupils

    C   It has been shown that after RK it is common for subjects to have steeper corneas in the afternoon than in the morning

    D   It has been shown that after RK some subjects are more myopic in the morning than in the afternoon

Visual optics: Answers

38 Item A is the only one which is correct, while the others tend to be the reverse of the truth.

References

Grosvenor, T. and Flom, M.C. (1991) *Refractive Anomalies*, Butterworth-Heinemann, Boston, pp. 135–145
Sorsby, A. and Leary, G.A. (1970) *A Longitudinal Study of Refraction and its Components During Growth*, HMSO, London, pp. 31–35
Van Alphen, G.W.H.M. (1990) In *Ciba Symposium 155: Myopia and the Control of Eye Growth*, Wiley, Chichester, pp. 115–125

39 Item C is the only correct pair of measurements. The radii involved correspond to powers of 45.00 D (337.5/7.50) and 41.00 D (337.5/8.23).

References

Douthwaite, W.A. (1987) *Contact Lens Optics*, Butterworths, London, p. 80
Phillips, A.J. and Stone, J. (eds) (1989) *Contact Lenses*, Butterworths. London, Appendix BP/910, Columns 1 and 9

40 Item C is the most likely one. Naturally, there are individual variations but the remaining items tend to express unusual rather than likely trends.

References

Bullimore, M. *et al.* (1994) Diurnal changes in radial keratotomy: implications for visual standards. *Optom and Vision Sci*, **B71**, 516–521
Easty, D. (1990) *Current Ophthalmic Surgery*, Baillière Tindall, London, pp. 243–244
van den Berg, J.T.P,. and IJspeert, J.K. (1992) Clinical assessment of intraocular stray light. *Applied Optics*, **32**, 3694–3696
Veraat, H.G. *et al.* (1992) Stray light in radial keratotomy and the influence of pupil size and straylight angle. *Am J Ophthalmol* **114**, 424–428
Walton, S.R. *et al.* (1988) *Surgery of the Eye*, Churchill Livingstone, Edinburgh, pp. 239–241

41 A reduced eye (refractive index 4/3) is 24 mm long. Without accommodating it receives a sharp retinal image of a vertical pin which is 25 mm high, placed 25 cm from the eye. Which one, or more, of the following is/are correct?

A   The radius of the ocular surface is 5.59 mm
B   The retinal image is inverted and is 0.8 mm in size
C   The retinal image is inverted and is 1.6 mm in size, while the radius of the ocular surface is 6.00 mm
D   The inverted retinal image is 1.8 mm in size

42 Ideas about the possible causes of myopia have included both environmental influences and inheritance. Much of the literature is ambiguous or lacks sustained conclusions but there are significant points which clinicians must consider. Which two of the following items are most likely to be the most significant guidance in practice?

A   Young's experiments with monkeys confined in small, bright spaces showed that in about a year the subjects developed marked 'refractive' myopia
B   Wiesel and Raviola produced monocular myopia in monkeys by depriving one eye of visual stimuli. This myopic change was found in young animals but not in adults
C   Accommodation, maintained for long periods in the absence of other contributory factors, is an important influence upon the development of myopia
D   Chicks wore a contact lens on one eye for 2 weeks. Eyes wearing +8.00 D lenses became relatively hyperopic; eyes wearing −10 D lenses became relatively myopic

Visual optics: Answers

41 Both items A and D are correct. A useful approach is with a diagram and simple calculations. Start with the refractive error, K, obviously −4.00 D when K = L. Also, L′ = K′, so K′ = (1000 × 4)/(24 × 3) = +55.55 D and F_e = K′ − K = +59.55 D. Using F = n'-n/r finding r = 5.59 mm h′ (retinal image) = h × L/L′ = −1.8 mm.

42 There could be some argument but the first two items, A and B, are probably the most helpful, even when compared to D. Item C is likely to be the opposite of many informed opinions.

References

Schaeffel, F., Glasser, A. and Howland, H.C. (1988) Accommodation, refractive error and eye growth in chickens. *Vision Res*, **28**, 639–657

Sivak, J.G. (1988) Reply to Birnbaum. *Am J Optom Physiol Optics*, **65**, 975 (re item C)

Wiesel, T.N. and Raviola, E. (1977) Myopia and eye enlargement after neonatal lid fusion in monkeys. *Nature*, March 3, 66–68

Young, F.A. (1961) The development and retention of myopia by monkeys. *Am J Optom Arch Am Acad Optom*, **38**, 545–555

43 A young emmetrope views a diapositive (transparency) monocularly. It is in the plane of a thin lens 'a', both being 20 cm from his eye. Midway between lens 'a' and the eye is a lens 'b', both lenses being +10.00 DS and thin. A point source of light is 10 cm beyond lens 'a'. Lens 'b' is then removed and the subject accommodates for the diapositive. Next, lens 'b' is replaced and lens 'a' is removed, the diapositive remaining in place. As a final arrangement, both lenses are placed in their original positions but the source is moved 5 cm so that it is 5 cm from lens 'a'. Which arrangement will give the highest illuminance to the retinal image of the diapositive?

A When the source is 5 cm from the diapositive and both lenses are used

B When only lens 'a' is used, with the source 10 cm from it

C When only lens 'b' is used, with the source 20 cm from it

D When the source is 10 cm from the diapositive and both lenses are used

44 A useful approach to understanding the formation of a retinal image in an eye corrected by a spectacle lens is to remember that the spectacle lens forms an image (h2) of a distant object (h), this image being in the plane of the far point. The eye is assumed to look at h2 and the eye forms a retinal image (h2′).

Consider a 'reduced' (single surface) eye which has an axial length of 25 mm and which is corrected for a distant object by a thin −10.00 DS lens placed 15 mm from the reduced surface. The eye has the standard refractive index of 4/3. Thus the spectacle Rx is −10.00 DS and the ocular refractive error (K) is −8.70 DS.

A distant object, which subtends 10 prism dioptres at the lens, is imaged sharply on the retina. Which of the following will be the correct size of the (inverted) retinal image (h2′)?

A −0.63 mm

B −1.63 mm

C −2.63 mm

D −3.63 mm

43 Item D should be chosen since this provides a 'Maxwellian view' and the source is imaged in the subject's pupil.

References

Fletcher, R. and Voke, J. (1985) *Defective Colour Vision*, Hilger, Bristol, pp. 514–515

Le Grand, Y. (1968) *Light, Colour and Vision*, 2nd edn, Chapman & Hall, London, pp. 102, 134 and 137

Wyszecki, G. and Stiles, W.S. (1982) *Color Science*, 2nd edn, John Wiley, New York, pp. 276, 479 and 481–482

44 Item B is correct. One approach is to consider that an image of the distant object (h2) which is formed in the plane of the far point, being 100 mm from the lens and subtending 10 prism dioptres, is 10 mm in size. The ocular refraction K is –8.70 DS and the vergence of light inside the eye, K', is related to the axial length (k') and the refractive index. Therefore $K' = 1000n'/k' = 4000/3 \times 25 = +53.33$ D. But $h2'/h2 = K/K'$, so $h2' = -870/+53.33 = -1.63$ mm.

When in doubt, draw a simple diagram.

References

Bennett, A.G. and Rabbetts, R.B. (1989) *Clinical Visual Optics*, 2nd edn, Butterworths, London, pp. 79–81

Obstfeld, H. (1982) *Optics in Vision*, 2nd edn, Butterworth Scientific, London, pp. 125–140

45 A hyperopic eye has its far point behind the eye in a virtual position. An image formed optically in this position acts as an object for the eye, which forms a sharp retinal image of appropriate size. Consider a 'reduced' (single surface) eye with a refractive index of 4/3, with a virtual image in its far point plane, which is 90 mm behind the refracting surface of the eye. The eye, which has a radius of curvature of +6.00 mm is then in focus for this virtual image and uses it as an object, forming a sharp retinal image. Select from the following list the correct axial length for the eye. You should recall that a 'standard' reduced eye has a radius of curvature of 50/9 mm and a length of 22.22 mm and consider the possibility that the eye you are considering may be axially hyperopic! Using the vergence reaching the ocular surface and the power of the eye, determine the correct axial length.

A   19.85 mm
B   20.00 mm
C   20.15 mm
D   20.30 mm

46 Many theories have been proposed about causes of myopia. One attributes myopia, among other refractive errors, to the variability and chance combinations of the optical elements of the eye which are chiefly inherited. Which of the following refers to this point of view?

A   Adolf Steiger's theory
B   Stilling's theory
C   The duplicity theory
D   Verhoeff's theory

45 Item B is correct. Because the power of the eye (Fe) = +55.56 D and the ocular refractive error (K) = K′, the vergence inside the eye, Fe + K = K′ = +66.67 D. Then the axial length (k′) which is the image space distance = $1000n'/66.67$ mm = +20 mm.

References

Bennett, A.G. and Rabbetts, R.B. (1989) *Clinical Visual Optics*, 2nd edn, Butterworths, London, pp. 74–75

Obstfeld, H. (1982) *Optics in Vision*, 2nd edn, Butterworth Scientific, London, pp. 71–73

46 Item A is correct. A. Steiger, a Swiss ophthalmologist, published his work in Berlin in 1913. Stilling related myopia to extraocular muscle action and intraocular pressure. The duplicity and Verhoeff's theory are not related to myopia.

References

Cline, D., Hofstetter, H.W. and Griffin, J.R. (1989) *Dictionary of Visual Science*, 4th edn, Chilton Trade, Radnor, pp. 748–749

Duke-Elder, W.S. (1949) *Textbook of Ophthalmology*, IV, Kimpton, London, p. 4339

Duke-Elder, W.S. (1970) *System of Ophthalmology*, V, Kimpton, London, pp. 241–242

47 Ultraviolet radiation of wavelength 300 nm is within the spectral band known as UV-B. Any consideration of ocular effects of such radiation should involve the transmittance of the ocular media and of lenses or filters which might give protection. Which of the following is most likely to be correct?

A   The action spectrum for UV-B has a higher threshold (for radiant exposure) than the threshold for UV-A at 350 nm

B   There are no types of intraocular implants which absorb UV radiation in order to protect the retina in pseudophakia

C   Crown glass transmits less radiation of 300 nm wavelength than is transmitted by a lens of polycarbonate of the same thickness

D   A polycarbonate lens absorbs more UV-B than is absorbed by a lens of crown glass of the same thickness

Visual optics: Answers

47 Item D is the only correct one. Various types of IOL have properties which block UV.

References

McKinlay, A.F., Harlen, F. and Whillock, M.J. (1988) *Hazards of Optical Radiation*, Hilger, Bristol, pp. 19–23

Miller, D. (1987) *Clinical Light Damage to the Eye*, Springer, New York, p. 148

Pitts, D.G. (1981) Threat of ultraviolet radiation to the eye – how to protect against it. *J Am Optom Ass*, 52, 949–957

Pitts, D.G. and Kleinstein, R.N. (1993) *Environmental Vision*, Butterworth-Heinemann, Boston, pp. 88, 166 and 274

48 The level of luminance of an optotype influences visual acuity
with fixation at and near the fovea. Some patients have
'eccentric fixation' following disturbances of foveal function;
clinical interpretation can be assisted by measurements at
different levels of optotype luminance. Figure 1.10 has been
developed from data by Sloan (1968) and shows slopes
according to the locations of fixation by a normal subject.
Which of the following is most likely to be a correct
interpretation, since the three lines are not identified in the
Figure?

A The top line, marked A, refers to fixation which gives a
retinal image 2 degrees from the fovea; line B refers to
10 degrees eccentricity while line C refers to foveal fixation

B Line A refers to fixation giving a retinal image 2 degrees
from the fovea, line C to an image at 10 degrees eccentricity
and line B refers to foveal fixation

C Line A refers to foveal fixation, line B to an image
2 degrees from the fovea and line C to an image
10 degrees from the fovea

D Line A refers to a retinal image 10 degrees from the fovea,
line B to one which is displaced 2 degrees from the fovea
and line C refers to an image on the fovea

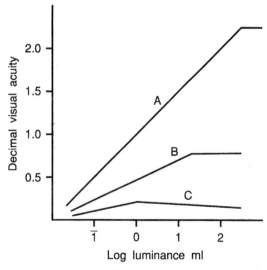

Fig. 1.10 Possible variations of visual acuity with changes in
luminance.

Visual optics: Answers

48 Item C is the correct one.

References

Davson, H. (1990) *Physiology of the Eye*, 5th edn, Macmillan, London, pp. 373–374 and 380

Randall, H.G., Brown, D.J. and Sloan, L.L. (1966) Peripheral visual acuity. *Arch Ophthalmol*, **75**, 500–504

Sloan, L.L. (1968) The photopic acuity–luminance function with special reference to parafoveal vision. *Vision Res*, **8**, 901–911

49 Laser radiation has been used for several ocular surgical methods, the choice of the most appropriate wavelength for a particular purpose being a matter of some debate. There are other non-surgical but surgery-related uses for lasers connected with the eye. Which two of the following are most likely to be correct?

A Grid patterns can be seen by cataractous patients when a system of low-power laser interferometry is applied to their eyes. Estimates of potential visual acuity can be made, although these may be overoptimistic

B A laser operating at wavelengths in the ultraviolet ranges would be most suitable for photocoagulation, where absorption by haemoglobin or the pigment epithelium is needed

C The argon laser, with a wavelength about 500 nm, or a krypton laser, with a wavelength between 641 and 647 nm, would be absorbed by pigment in the eye, with the argon type likely to have less effect on the choroid

D An ideal laser for retinal therapy would be one which is badly absorbed by the retinal pigment epithelium

50 Sunglasses or other forms of protective eyewear use lenses which obey the basic laws which apply to filters generally. Which two of the following suggestions are correct?

A Suppose that a certain glass lens which is 4.6 mm thick, acting as a filter to light with a wavelength of 500 nm, has a spectral transmission factor of 48 per cent. This factor will be approximately doubled if the thickness is reduced to 2 mm

B Light flux entering a normal glass filter at a slight angle passes through and emerges. The light flux emerging has been reduced from the original value only by absorption

C The spectral transmittance of a series of filters, all separated by air, is given by the product of the spectral transmittances of the individual filters

D According to British Standard 7394: Part 2: (1994) which concerns 'complete spectacles', a 'luminous transmission factor' (as a percentage) is higher for a 'medium' photochromic lens than for an 'extra dark' photochromic lens

49 Items A and C are most likely. The excimer laser (approximately 160–350 nm) is used for corneal surgery. Most retinal procedures aim at good absorption by the pigment epithelium.

References
Anonymous editorial. (1979) Search for the ideal laser. *Br J Ophthalmol*, **63**, 655–656

Ariffin, A., Hill, R.D. and Leigh, O. (1992) *Diabetes and Primary Eye Care*, Blackwell Scientific, Oxford, p. 111

L'Esperance, F.A. (1990) Ophthalmic lasers: current status. In *Ophthalmic Surgery*, 2nd edn (ed. G.L. Spaeth), Saunders, Philadelphia, pp. 113–119 (see also p. 130)

Pitts, D.G. and Kleinstein, R.N. (1993) *Environmental Vision*, Butterworth-Heinemann, Boston, p. 229

50 Items C and D are the correct ones.

References
BS 7394: Part 2: (1994) British Standards Institution, London

Jalie, M. (1975) Variations in transmission of a filter. *Ophthalmic Optician*, **15**, 135–136

Wyszecki, G. and Stiles, W.S. (1982) *Color Science*, 2nd edn, Wiley, New York, pp. 30–32

51 Working conditions influence visual performance in many ways. Various approaches to the evaluation of 'visual performance' have been attempted, in order to study the effects of different environmental and stimulus conditions which apply at work or during driving or sporting activities. Which two of the following are *incorrect*?

A The proportion of errors made when undertaking inspection of woven fabrics in a factory is usually found to increase as the intensity of illuminance increases

B The 'conspicuity area' of a briefly presented target whose location is unknown is part of the visual field which is usually smaller than the 'visibility area', since the latter involves attention

C At a target contrast of 25 per cent, with decimal visual acuity at 1.0 when background luminance is about 340 cd/m^2, the decimal visual acuity would probably be 0.01 with a background luminance of 3.4 cd/m^2

D Assuming that reading a typical book involves ink which reflects about 4 per cent of incident light, on paper reflecting 80 per cent, the contrast is about 95 per cent

52 A plane mirror effect self-luminous retinoscope is constructed. Two lenses are placed between the source and the sighthole, which are 11 cm apart. One lens, a, is placed 5 cm from the source and the other, b, is placed half way between lens a and the sighthole. Light must leave the region of the sighthole with a vergence of about −0.75 D on its way to the patient. One lens is +15.00 DS, but is it a or b? What is the power of the other lens most likely to be?

A +7.75 DS
B −6.65 DS
C −0.75 DS
D +0.75 DS

Visual optics: Answers

51 Items A and C are the incorrect items. Errors tend to decrease with significant increases in illuminance, correctly applied. The decrease in visual acuity is likely to be from 1.0 to only 0.50.

References
Blackwell, H.R. (1946) Contrast thresholds of the human eye. *J Opt Soc Am*, **36**, 624–643
Donk, M. (1993) On the comparison of conspicuity with visibility. In *Visual Search 2* (ed. D. Brogan *et al.*), Taylor & Francis, London, pp. 333–339
Duke-Elder, W.S. and Abrams, D. (1970) *System of Ophthalmology*, V, Kimpton, London, pp. 583–589
Pitts, D.G. and Kleinstein, R.N. (1993) *Environmental Vision*, Butterworth-Heinemann, Boston, p. 119
Weston, H.C. (1944) Brightness, well-being and work. *Br J Indust Med*, **1**, 181–196

52 It is logical to place a high power 'condensing' lens nearest to the source and it is 'a', which should be the +15.00 DS lens. A second lens of power given in item B would be most likely to provide the necessary retinoscopic beam.

53 Trial case lenses are generally assumed to be thin, and thus may be simply added together to determine the *back vertex power*. This is not, however, the case, particularly with higher powered corrections. Additive vertex power sets have therefore been designed in an attempt to simplify prescribing. Which of the following statements concerning the use of such sets is *incorrect*?

    A   Cylinders must be placed in the back cell with the toric surface nearest the eye

    B   In the absence of a cylindrical correction a *plano* lens must be placed in the trial frame

    C   The spheres must be biconvex or biconcave in form

    D   The power marked on the spheres will not be exactly the same as that found if they are measured on a focimeter

54 Which of the following formulae does *not* relate to contrast sensitivity measurement?

    A $y = a\sin(bx) + c$

    B $\text{Modulation} = \dfrac{L_{max} - L_{min}}{L_{max} + L_{min}}$

    C $\text{Luminance contrast} = \left(\dfrac{L_1 - L_2}{L_1}\right) \times 100\%$

    D   Spatial frequency $v = 1/\theta$ cycles/degree

Visual optics: Answers

53 C is incorrect. The lenses must have flat back surfaces. This ensures that when the lenses are correctly positioned in the trial frame, with the spheres in front of the cylinders (plano surfaces facing each other), the distance separating the lenses is constant, regardless of the powers involved. As long as the cylindrical lenses are of equal thickness, the back vertex powers may be determined by simple addition of the marked values. The value marked on the spheres is that of the effective power at the cylindrical surface, and thus may differ slightly to the power when measured by focimeter.

References
Bennett, A.G. (1968) *Emsley and Swaine's Ophthalmic Lenses*, Hatton Press, London, pp. 170–179

BS 3162 (1989) *Specification for Ophthalmic Trial Case Lenses*, British Standards Institution, Milton Keynes (this suggested an alternative to the additive vertex power approach, with flat lenses whose plano surfaces could be adjacent, placing the curved surfaces of spherical lenses nearest to the eye)

Jalie, M. (1984) *The Principles of Ophthalmic Lenses*, 4th edn, Association of Dispensing Opticians, London, pp. 352–358

54 The correct response, C, refers to contrast on a standard letter chart in which the area of the black lettering is different to the area of white background. If L_1 is the luminance of the white background of a test chart and L_2 the luminance of the black lettering, then formula C is used to determine if the standard test chart requirement of 90% contrast (BS 4274 1968) has been reached. It should be noted that BS 4274 is now obsolete; however, no alternative Standard has been devised.

Formula A refers to the standard formula for a sine curve, B to the modulation of luminance of a sine wave and D to the spatial frequency of a sine wave; thus are all relevant to contrast sensitivity measurement.

References
Bennett, A.G. and Rabbetts, R.B. (1989) *Clinical Visual Optics*, 2nd edn, Butterworths, London, pp. 40–41

BS 4274 (1968) *Test Charts for Determining Visual Acuity*, British Standards Institution, Milton Keynes

Tunnacliff, A.H. (1984) *Introduction to Visual Optics*, Association of Dispensing Opticians, London, pp. 379 and 407–409

55 Visual acuity may be expressed in several ways. If visual acuity has been noted as logMAR 0.6 (where MAR is the minimum angle of resolution), which of the following equivalent values is *incorrect*?

A Decimal acuity = 0.6
B Snellen (metric) = 6/24
C Snellen (feet) = 20/80
D Minimum angle of resolution = 4 min of arc

56 A logical way of designing test charts is to use a geometrical progression in which each line is a precise amount larger than the previous line. Which geometrical progression is used in the design of the Bailey Lovie test chart?

A Each row is 1.2589 times the size of the previous one
B Each row is 1.2599 times the size of the previous one
C Each row is 1.4142 times the size of the previous one
D Each row is 1.4678 times the size of the previous one

55 A is incorrect, being equal to logMAR 0.2, 6/10 and 20/33. As decimal acuity is equal to the reciprocal of the minimum angle of resolution (MAR), it is necessary to find the antilog value for 0.6 (i.e. 4) and then take its reciprocal (i.e. 1/4 = 0.25). Alternatively, decimal acuity is found by dividing the test distance by the letter size (i.e. the reciprocal of minimum angle of resolution); in this case the answer would be 0.25.

References
Bennett, A.G. and Rabbetts, R.B. (1989) *Clinical Visual Optics*, 2nd edn, Butterworths, London, p. 32

Farrall, H. (1991) *Optometric Management of Visual Handicap*, Blackwell Scientific, Oxford, pp. 38–42

Lovie-Kitchin, J.E. and Bowman, K.J. (1985) *Senile Macular Degeneration*, Butterworths, Boston, pp. 60–63

56 A is used by the Bailey Lovie chart, this being chosen so that the 10th row is 10 times larger than the 1st. Answer B is the cube root of 2, thus the letter size doubles every 3rd row, C is the square root of 2 which would cause the letter size to double every 2nd row, and D is the 6th root of 10, which causes the letter size to increase ten fold after 6 rows and approximates to the progression used in the standard Snellen charts.

References
Bennett, A.G. and Rabbetts, R.B. (1989) *Clinical Visual Optics*, 2nd edn, Butterworths, London, p. 32

Farrall, H. (1991) *Optometric Management of Visual Handicap*, Blackwell Scientific, Oxford, pp. 38–42

Lovie-Kitchin, J.E. and Bowman, K.J. (1985) *Senile Macular Degeneration*, Butterworths, Boston, pp. 60–63

Sloan, L.L. (1959) New test for the measurement of visual acuity at far and near distances. *Am J Ophthalmol*, **55**, p. 1187

57 A point source of white light is placed at the anterior focal point of a positive lens, through which a subject sees the light. Which one of the following best describes the effect of viewing this white light source through both holes of a Scheiner disc placed in front of the eye with the holes vertical to one another and the upper hole covered by a red filter?

A   A myopic eye will see a double image, with a red upper image

B   A non-accommodating hyperopic eye will see a double image, with a red upper image

C   A single image will be seen regardless of the refractive error of the eye

D   A double image will be seen regardless of the refractive error of the eye

58 A phoropter (refractor head) has a ±0.50 DC crossed cylinder lens (minus axis vertical) which may be used in conjunction with a test card consisting of horizontal and vertical lines, for the determination of reading adds. Assuming the patient (wearing full distance correction) reports that, at his normal viewing distance, the vertical lines are clearer, which one of the following statements is most likely to be true?

A   The reading add is too weak

B   A decrease in the add is required

C   No change in add is required

57 A is the correct answer. Remember that retinal images are projected into space through the eye's nodal point, thus the inverted retinal image will be seen upright. Figure 1.11 shows that although a myopic eye will receive light passing through the upper hole on the lower part of the retina, it will be perceived as the higher (red) image.

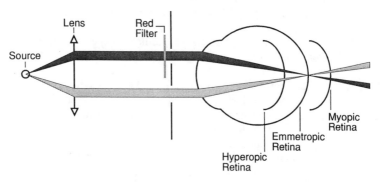

Fig. 1.11 Collimated light reaching retina through Scheiner disc with one hole covered with red filter.

Reference

Bennett, A.G. and Rabbetts, R.B. (1989) *Clinical Visual Optics*, 2nd edn, Butterworths, London

58 B is true. The crossed cylinder for reading add determination is orientated (on a refractor head) such that the minus axis is vertical. This will induce 'with-the-rule' astigmatism in which the back focal line is vertical. If excessive plus power is added, the vertical lines will lie closer to the retina, causing them to appear clearer.

References

Bennett, A.G. and Rabbetts, R.B. (1989) *Clinical Visual Optics*, 2nd edn, Butterworths, London, p. 144

Borish, I.M. (1970) *Clinical Refraction*, 3rd edn, Professional Press, Chicago, pp. 181 and 841

Woo, G.C. and Sivak, J.G. (1987) In *Presbyopia* (eds L. Stark and G. Obrecht), Professional Press, New York, pp. 310–312

59 If the spectacle correction, worn at a vertex distance of 12 mm, is −14.00/+3.00 × 90, what is the correction (to the nearest 0.12 D) at the cornea?

A   −12.00 DS/+3.00 DC × 90
B   −16.87 DS/+4.12 DC × 90
C   −12.00 DS/+2.25 DC × 90
D   −16.87 DS/+3.00 DC × 90

60 One of the problems solved by the use of intraocular lens implants is the reduced field of vision caused by the spectacle correction of aphakics. However, it is still occasionally necessary to correct an aphakic with spectacles. Such a correction results in a loss of field, resulting in the 'Jack-in-the-box' effect whereby objects jump in or out of the field of view. Assuming an aphake has a correction of +14 DS worn 25 mm from the eye's centre of rotation, which of the following represents the annulus of field loss in a spherical lenticular of diameter 40 mm?

A   14°
B   16°
C   22°
D   32°

59 C is correct. At the cornea, the more myopic principal meridian −14 becomes (to the nearest 0.25 D) −12.00 DS, the less myopic meridian (−11 at 12 mm) becomes −9.75 DS, thus the ocular refraction would be −12.00 DS/+2.25 DC × 90 (to the nearest 0.25 D).

References
Bennett, A.G. (1985) *Optics of Contact Lens*, 3rd edn, Association of Dispensing Opticians, London, pp. 7 and 89

Douthwaite, W.A. (1987) *Contact Lens Optics*, Butterworths, London, pp. 1–3

60 C is correct (Figure 1.12).

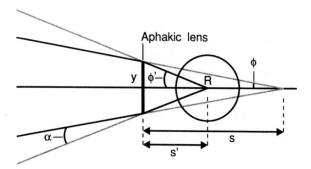

Fig. 1.12 The effect of a spectacle correction on the aphake's visual field. y = semi-diameter of the lens; s′ = distance from lens to centre of rotation (R); s = distance from lens to image of centre of rotation; 2φ = real field of view; 2φ′ = apparent field of view; α = annulus of field loss.

If a lens of power +14, aperture = 40 mm (y = 20 mm), and s′ = 25 mm, then

$$\tan \phi = 20*(40-14)/1000 = 20*26/1000 = 0.52$$

Thus $\phi = 27.5°$, giving a real field of view of 55° instead of a field of view of 77.3° ($\tan^{-1}$ ($^{20}/_{25}$) = $\tan^{-1}$ 0.8 = 38.66° for half the field of view). The annulus (α) of field loss is thus 77 − 55°, or 22° in size. This calculation assumes the eye is in the primary position and does not consider the effect of spherical aberrations, etc. in reducing field of vision.

Reference
Jalie, M. (1984) *The Principles of Ophthalmic Lenses*, 4th edn, Association of Dispensing Opticians, London, pp. 115–119

2 Clinical techniques

1 In automated 'static threshold' perimetry, a Goldmann III
(4 mm^2) type stimulus can be used on a Humphrey field analyser.
When this is done, using an intensity of 20 decibels (dB), which
of the following statements applies?

A Seeing the stimulus indicates greater sensitivity than when
   threshold is at 10 dB
B The 20 dB stimulus has a greater luminance than one of
   10 dB
C The Humphrey stimulus of 20 dB is exactly the same as a
   20 dB 'Octopus' type stimulus
D The 20 dB 'Humphrey' stimulus is more readily seen than
   one of 40 dB

2 The Amsler grid (held at distances sometimes said to be 28 cm,
sometimes 35 cm) is a useful clinical test of part of the visual
field, including apparent distortions. Which of the following
regions of the retina is most likely to be evaluated, using the
grid?

A Approximately 10 degrees, in all directions, measured from
   the fovea
B Only the centrocaecal region, involving the papillomacular
   fibres
C Approximately 1.75 prism dioptres in all directions, from the
   fovea
D A square region extending a total of about 10 degrees with its
   centre on the optic disc

2 Clinical techniques: Answers

1 D is the one which applies. For the Humphrey instrument 20 dB represent 100 asb but 40 dB represent only 1 asb, hence the stronger stimulus has an advantage. The Humphrey system uses the relationship

$$1\,dB = 10 \times \log (10\,000\,asb)$$

The Octopus system uses

$$1\,dB = 10 \times \log (1000\,asb)$$

The decibel value is proportional to sensitivity.

References

Eskridge, B. *et al.* (1991) *Clinical Procedures in Optometry*, Lippincott, Philadelphia, p. 449
Krupin, T. (1988) *Manual of Glaucoma*, Churchill Livingstone, New York, p. 62
Townsend, J.C. *et al.* (1991) *Visual Fields*, Butterworth-Heinemann, Boston, p. 25

2 Item A is the one which applies. The standard form of grid has 20 × 20 squares, each of 5 mm, each subtending approximately 1 degree. Note that, assuming that 7 prism dioptres represent 4 degrees and 1.75 represent 1 degree, the area suggested in C is much too small.

References

Eskridge, B. *et al.* (1991) *Clinical Procedures in Optometry*, Lippincott, Philadelphia, p. 436
Faye, E.E. (1984) *Clinical Low Vision*, 2nd edn, Little, Brown, Boston, pp. 55–59
Miller, S. (1987) *Clinical Ophthalmology*, Butterworth Scientific, London, p. 322
Newman, N.M. (1992) *Neuro-Ophthalmology*, Appleton & Lange, Norwalk, Connecticut, p. 49
Rosenbloom, A.A. and Morgan, M.W. (1993) *Vision and Aging*, 2nd edn, Butterworth-Heinemann, Boston, p. 214
Townsend, J.C. *et al.* (1991) *Visual Fields*, Butterworth-Heinemann, Boston, p. 4

3 The term *drusen* is applied to certain yellowish, usually round, spots of discoloration mostly found in the central macular region of the fundus. Which of the following items is most likely to be *incorrect*?

  A Drusen distort the retinal surface of the retinal pigment epithelium
  B Drusen are essentially areas of severe thinning of Bruch's membrane
  C Drusen can be associated with age-related degeneration of the region
  D The term is derived from 'accumulation of crystals' in the German language
  E Drusen are usually found in each eye and are often symmetrically located

4 Migraine is found widely and in several forms. Which of the following items are most likely to be correct?

  A The onset of migraine is seldom at an age greater than 40 years
  B Scintillating scotomata are reported in all types of migraine
  C The term is not related to 'hemi' cranial features
  D There is a strong hereditary basis for the conditions described as migraine
  E The typical causes of migraine are associated by arterial dilatation followed by a phase of vasoconstriction

5 One fairly common form of optic disc, seen ophthalmoscopically, is described as a *tilted disc* and it has been said to be a congenital abnormality which has some clinical importance. Which two of the following items are most likely to be correct?

  A The condition may be associated with bitemporal visual field defects
  B It is never associated with situs inversus, in which the temporal vessels start in a nasal direction
  C There is likely to be an association with abnormal closure of the embryonic (choroidal) fissure
  D There is never any related decrement of visual acuity, such as might possibly be attributable to the Stiles–Crawford effect

Clinical techniques: Answers

3 Item B is *incorrect* and should have been chosen. Drusen are typically associated with diffuse thickening of Bruch's membrane in an area where retinal pigment epithelium cells, which lie over the drusen, become hypopigmented. The deposits have been described as comprising mucopolysaccharides and lipids, are often found in age-related degeneration of the region and are frequently bilateral and symmetrically distributed.

References

Freeman, W.R. (1993) *Practical Atlas of Retinal Disease and Therapy*, Raven Press, New York, pp. 155–157

Lovie-Kitchin, J.E. and Bowman, K.J. (1985) *Senile Macular Degeneration*, Butterworths, Boston and London, pp. 35–38

Scuderi, G. *et al.* (1987) *Atlas of Clinical Ophthalmoscopy*, Year Book, Chicago, pp. 76 and 164

4 A and D are most correct. In most populations the onset peaks between puberty and 30 years of age. It is only in the 'classical' type of migraine that scintillating scotomata are reported and therefore probably in less than 50% of patients with some sort of migraine. Most patients appear to have near relatives similarly affected. Extracranial blood flow tends to be greater during later (headache) phases, with, for example, dilated scalp arteries; cerebral blood flow is less during early stages.

References

Dalesso, D.J. (1987) *Wolff's Headache and Other Head Pains*, 5th edn, Oxford UP, Oxford, pp. 58–79

Newman, N.M. (1992) *Neuro-Ophthalmology*, Appleton & Lange, Norwalk, Connecticut, p. 310

Sandler, M. and Collins, G.M. (1990) *Migraine: A Spectrum of Ideas*, Oxford UP, Oxford, pp. 5–13, 95 and 191

5 Items A and C are correct. The incidence is about 2% and the condition is usually bilateral. The likely association with situs inversus, where the initial nasal course from the disc of the temporal vessels is notable, is possibly accompanied with a mimicry of bitemporal hemianopia. Slight lowering of visual acuity is sometimes found, with possibly amblyopia in monocular instances; the Stiles–Crawford effect may be involved.

References

Brown, G.C. and Tasman, W.S. (1983) *Congenital Anomalies of the Optic Disc*, Grune & Stratton, New York, pp. 86–87

Kritzinger, E.E. and Beaumont, H.M. (1987) *A Colour Atlas of Optic Disc Abnormalities*, Wolfe Medical, London, p. 24

Trachimowicz, R.A. (1994) Review of embryology and its relation to ocular disease in the pediatric population. *Optometry and Vision Science*, **71**, 162

6 Figure 2.1 shows records obtained from two subjects (a and b) using a certain conventional test method. Scale I indicates cycles per degree and scale II (vertical) shows contrast sensitivity. Which of the following items is the only one which is correct?

    A   Both scales indicate the spatial frequency of each stimulus presented

    B   If each subject is 'normal', the data for b are likely to be related to a higher retinal illuminance than those for a

    C   The point × on scale II indicates a greater sensitivity to contrast than point g

    D   The point × on scale II indicates that more contrast is needed than at point g

    E   Neither scale is likely to be plotted logarithmically

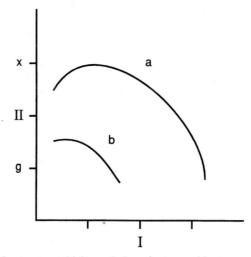

Fig. 2.1 Contrast sensitivity variations for two subjects.

6 Only item C is correct. Thus the sensitivity of subject a, given equal test conditions, would be seen as greater than that of subject b, for most frequencies.

References

Bennett, A.G. and Rabbetts, R.B. (1989) *Clinical Visual Optics*, 2nd edn, Butterworths, London, p. 62

DeValois, R.L. and DeValois, K.K. (1988) *Spatial Vision*, Oxford University Press, p. 151

Eskridge, J.B. (1991) *Clinical Procedures in Optometry*, Lippincott, Philadelphia, p. 499

Leigh, O. (1992) In *Diabetes and Primary Eye Care* (eds A. Ariffin *et al.*), Blackwell Scientific, Oxford, pp. 140–144

Nadler, M.P. *et al.* (1990) *Glare and Contrast Sensitivity for Clinicians*, Springer, New York, p. 127

Proenza, L.M., Enoch, J.M. and Jampolsky, A. (1981) *Clinical Applications of Visual Psychophysics*, Cambridge University Press, p. 25

7   Which of the following suggestions relating to the 'cover' test is *least* likely?

   A   The subjective cover test is useful in the detection of small angles of strabismus
   B   It is useful to repeat the cover test above and below the primary position of gaze in the detection of 'A' and 'V' patterns of incomitancy
   C   Figure 2.2 suggests that the patient (shown five times) has a left convergent strabismus
   D   An amblyopic esotropic eye with VA 6/60 should very rapidly take up fixation when the other (good) eye is occluded

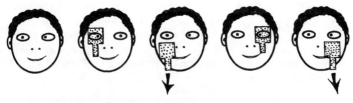

Fig. 2.2   Cover test sequence showing ocular movements.

8   Von Seidel's sign is a classical feature of at least one eye condition. In this connection, which of the following items is correct?

   A   It is otherwise described as a bitemporal hemianopia
   B   It is an extension of the blind spot, possibly at the top, which is rare in open angle glaucoma
   C   It is miosis caused by damage to the superior cervical ganglion
   D   It is an afferent pupil effect or related to jaw movement and otherwise associated with the same Marcus Gunn

Clinical techniques: Answers

7 As shown by Pickwell (1984) (using a slightly different situation), item C is not the least likely choice here; the situation might be less clear if eccentric fixation were to be involved. Item D should be chosen as least likely.

References
Daum, K.M. (1991) In *Clinical Procedures in Optometry* (eds J.B. Eskridge *et al.*), Lippincott, Philadelphia, pp. 73–80

Pickwell, D. (1984) *Binocular Vision Anomalies*, Butterworths, London, p. 15

Stidwill, D. (1990) *Orthoptic Assessment and Management*, Blackwell Scientific, Oxford, pp. 54–55

8 Von Seidel's sign is described by Brown, in Brown and Fletcher (1990), as a 'tapering extension' of the blind spot. In Dunbar *et al.* (1989) the term Seidel scotoma is used. Item A is incorrect. Item C is associated with Horner's syndrome while D is incorrect; for each of these, the Marcus Gunn pupil as well as the Marcus Gunn (jaw-winking) lid situation see Spalton *et al.* (1984). In addition, Nauman and Apple (1986) describe Horner's syndrome.

References
Brown, F.G. and Fletcher, R. (1990) *Glaucoma in Optometric Practice*, Blackwell Scientific, Oxford, pp. 160–161

Dunbar, Hoskins and Kass (1989) *Diagnosis and Therapy of the Glaucomas*, Mosby, St Louis, p. 142

Nauman, G.O.H. and Apple, D.J. (1986) *Pathology of the Eye*, Springer, New York, p. 423

Spalton, D.J. *et al.* (1984) *Atlas of Clinical Ophthalmology*, Churchill Livingstone, Edinburgh

9 Decimal fractions are used in some countries to describe vision or visual acuity as measured with optotypes. This method can be related to other descriptions so that 1.00 corresponds to 6/6 or 20/20 or log MAR (minimum angle of resolution) 0.00, all corresponding to a visual angle of 1.00 minute of arc. Which of the following corresponds to a visual angle of 2.00 minutes of arc?

A   log MAR 0.30
B   log MAR 1.00
C   6/9
D   20/15

10 There are many tests which involve the use of dots. Which test in the following list does not require the use of filters, such as are worn in polarizing or coloured spectacles or clip-on attachments?

A   The Worth four dot test
B   The Lang stereotest
C   The Titmus stereotest
D   The Randot stereotest
E   The Mallett fixation disparity test

11 Contrast sensitivity can be assessed by using 'low or variable' visual acuity tests or optotypes, as described by Bailey (1993) and others, or by displays of gratings. Which two of the following do *not* use letters or representations of a face?

A   Pelli–Robson chart
B   Regan low-contrast charts
C   Arden test
D   Cambridge test

9   Since log MAR 1.00 corresponds to an angle of 10 minutes, 6/9 to 1.5 minutes and 20/15 to 0.75 minutes, item A is correct.

References

Bennett, A.G. and Rabbetts, R.B. (1989) *Clinical Visual Optics*, 2nd edn, Butterworths, London, p. 36

Lovie-Kitchin, J.E. and Bowman, K.J. (1985) *Senile Macular Degeneration,* Butterworth, Boston, p. 62

10   As described by Stidwill (1990), the Lang test should be chosen here. All the others require filters.

References

Bennett, A.G. and Rabbetts, R.B. (1989) *Clinical Visual Optics*, Butterworths, London, pp. 241–243

Buckingham, T. (1993) *Visual Problems in Childhood*, Butterworth-Heinemann, Oxford, p. 216

Cooper, J. (1991) In *Clinical Procedures in Optometry* (eds J.B. Eskridge *et al.*), Lippincott, Philadelphia, pp. 121–134

Mein, J. and Trimble, R. (1986) *Diagnosis and Management of Ocular Motility Disorders*, 2nd edn, Blackwell Scientific, Oxford, pp. 139–141

Pratt-Johnson, J.A. and Tillson, G. (1994) *Management of Strabismus and Amblyopia*, Thieme, New York, p. 39

Stidwill, D. (1990) *Orthoptic Assessment and Management*, Blackwell Scientific, Oxford, p. 26

11   The last two items are correct as they use different forms of gratings.

References

Arden, G.B. and Jacobson, J.J. (1978) A simple grating test for contrast sensitivity. *Invest Ophthalmol Vis Sci*, **17**, 23

Bailey, I.L. (1993) New procedures for detecting early vision losses in the elderly. *Optometry and Vision Science*, **70**, 299–305

Nadler, M.P. *et al.* (1990) *Glare and Contrast Sensitivity for Clinicians*, Springer, New York, pp. 37–43

Thompson, C. (1993) In *Visual Problems in Childhood* (ed. T. Buckingham), Butterworth-Heinemann, Oxford, pp. 181–184

12 The need for appropriate spectral distribution of energy when illuminating most colour vision tests is recognized. Which of the following is the most suitable level of illuminance, for tests using Munsell colour samples, assuming correct orientation of the test and a proper viewing distance?

A 10 lux
B 5000 lux
C 100–600 lux
D 7500 lux

13 A patient alleges that one eye is blind. You place a prism, base horizontal, in front of this eye and a definite fusional movement results. The best objective correction is in place. Which of the following suggestions is most likely to be correct?

A Visual acuity in the bad eye is worse than 6/80
B The eye is blind
C It is unlikely that visual acuity in the 'blind' eye can be improved in any way
D Visual acuity in the 'blind' eye is at least 6/60

14 Sloan's charts used for near visual evaluation use M units and can assist in the measurement of near corrected acuity and reading ability. Which of the following is the only correct statement?

A Capital letters only are used
B Capital letters are used as well as sections of continuous text
C Numbers only are used, in equal logarithmic steps
D Text using only lower case letters is used

12 According to Bowman and Cole (1980) with respect to the Farnsworth–Munsell 100 hue test, there is little point in using over 100 lux, at least for young subjects. It was for 100 lux that Verriest's 'norms' were stated. There is a likelihood of tritan type errors tending to be found below 20 lux.

References

Bowman, K. and Cole, B.L. (1980) *Am J Optom Physiol Opt*, **57**, 839–843

Chioran, G.M. and Sheedy, J.E. (1983) Pseudoisochromatic plate design – Macbeth or tungsten illumination. *Am J Optom Physiol Opt*, **60**, 204–215

Fletcher, R. and Voke, J. (1985) *Defective Colour Vision*, Hilger, Bristol, pp. 268 and 302

Pokorny, J., Smith, V.C. *et al.* (1979) *Congenital and Acquired Color Vision Defects*, Grune & Stratton, New York, pp. 103–106

13 It is reasonable to select D, although it would also be reasonable to add at least one or two extra malingering tests.

References

Allen, R.J., Fletcher, R. and Still, D.C. (1991) *Eye Examination and Refraction*, Blackwell Scientific, Oxford, pp. 132–134 and 207–208

Duke-Elder, W.S. (1970) *System of Ophthalmology*, Kimpton, London, pp. 487–501

14 Item B is the correct one. Sloan's charts for use at 40 cm use capitals, which are varied in size in equal steps on a logarithmic scale. Reading ability is tested with her reading cards using text also arranged in M units.

References

Farrall, H. (1991) *Optometric Management of Visual Handicap*, Blackwell Scientific, Oxford, pp. 45–49

Faye, E.E. (1984) *Clinical Low Vision*, 2nd edn, Little, Brown, Boston, pp. 47–51

Sloan, L.L. (1977) *Reading Aids for the Partially Sighted*, Williams & Wilkins, Baltimore, pp. 44–50

15 A patient can just read 3M size print (=N18) at 40 cm, using conventional reading lenses (incorporating a +2.50 D addition) but needs more plus power to be able to read 1 M size print (=N5), albeit at a suitably adjusted distance. Which of the following suggestions is this extra power most likely to be?

A   Between +7.50 and +9.75 D
B   Between +25 and +34 D
C   Between +17.50 and +24 D
D   Between +3.75 and +4.75 D

16 It is well recognized that many 'acquired' colour vision deficiencies are manifested by 'tritan' type confusions. Which of the following tests is the only one to include pseudoisochromatic (PIC) plates for detecting tritan errors?

A   Ishihara plates
B   Standard PIC plates (1978) (Part 1) Ichikawa, H. *et al.*, Igaku-Shoin, Tokyo
C   Ohkuma's test cards (1986) Kanehara, Tokyo
D   Standard PIC plates (1983) (Part 2) Ichikawa, H. *et al.*, Igaku-Shoin, Tokyo

17 Amplitude of accommodation and its measurement are important in clinical practice. In this connection, which of the following items is most likely to be correct?

A   An accelerated tendency to lowering of accommodation is sometimes found in juvenile diabetic patients
B   A tendency to show increased accommodation, not related to any miosis, is found in cases of glaucoma with ciliary body atrophy
C   When using dynamic retinoscopy to measure accommodative amplitude it is usual to find that early presbyopes need, for reading, about +1.00 DS more than the high neutral
D   A young subject with a high amplitude of accommodation must always be 'fogged' by at least +0.50 DS when measuring astigmatism with a crossed cylinder method

75

Clinical techniques: Answers

15 Item A is most likely to suit, although a trial would be needed. Various approaches are possible, such as noting that a magnification of some ×3 is needed which requires a total nominal plus addition of +12 D and, allowing for the original +2.50 D, that suggests an extra +9.50 D. A comparison of the references would indicate why the range in item A is given.

References
Bier, N. (1960) *Correction of Subnormal Vision*, Butterworths, London, p. 153
Farrall, H. (1991) *Optometric Management of Visual Handicap*, Blackwell Scientific, Oxford, p. 192 (for practical example)
Fonda, G. (1970) *Management of the Patient with Subnormal Vision*, 2nd edn, Mosby, Saint Louis, p. 136
Lovie-Kitchin, J.E. and Bowman, K.J. (1985) *Senile Macular Degeneration*, Butterworths, Boston, pp. 94–97

16 Item D, the Part 2 plates by Ichikawa *et al.* (1983) do include tritan plates as well as protan and deutan plates. The others only attempt to test for protan and deutan defects.

References
Fletcher, R. and Voke, J. (1985) *Defective Colour Vision*, Hilger, Bristol, pp. 281–282
Ichikawa, K., Ichikawa, H. and Tanabe, S. (1987) Detection of acquired color vision defects by standard pseudoisochromatic plates Part 2. In *Colour Vision Deficiencies* (ed. G. Verriest), VIII, Junk, Dordrecht, pp. 133–143

17 Item A is the correct one; see Ariffin *et al.* (1992). For the difficulty with item B, see Eskridge *et al.* (1991). Regarding the other two items see Allen *et al.* (1991).

References
Allen, R.J., Fletcher, R. and Still, D.C. (1991) *Eye Examination and Refraction*, Blackwell Scientific, Oxford, pp. 90 and 111
Ariffin, A., Hill, R.D. and Leigh, O. (1992) Blackwell Scientific, Oxford, pp. 61–62
Eskridge, J.B. *et al.* (1991) *Clinical Procedures in Optometry*, Lippincott, New York, p. 71
Whitefoot, H. and Charman, W.N. (1992) Dynamic retinoscopy and accommodation. *Ophthal Physiol Opt*, **12**, 8–17

18 When ophthalmoscopy is frustrated, by cataract or other opacity, ultrasonography is a valuable means of investigation; it is also frequently used before cataract surgery. Three of the following statements are unreliable; which of the four is the correct one?

A   It is not possible to detect a retinal detachment by the use of ultrasonography

B   A B-scan ultrasonogram is capable of demonstrating a total retinal detachment

C   The axial length of an eye, as measured by ultrasound, is greater than the 'optical' axial length because of a factor introduced by retinal thickness

D   There is considerable doubt about the adverse effects of the energy levels used for ocular diagnosis by ultrasound

19 A medical student is soon to start some involvement with Down's syndrome children and wishes to discuss with you the following matters. What are the types and the extent of visual handicap likely to be involved, therefore which tests are most useful? Which one of the following suggestions is correct and therefore useful as a start for the discussion?

A   Down's syndrome children are unlikely to have strabismus, so cover testing is hardly suitable

B   Myopia is present in over 60 per cent of such children but cataract is rare

C   Visual acuity and ocular motility in Down's syndrome children is likely to be no worse than in the general population in the same age group

D   Investigations differ as to the proportion of deutan or protan colour vision deficiency among Down's syndrome children, when compared to the general population but adequate test methods should show little difference

Clinical techniques: Answers

18 The misleading suggestions are A and D (see Fielding, 1994, pp. 94–95), also C (see Retzlaff *et al.*, 1990, p. 336). Therefore item B is correct (see, for example, Smith *et al.*, 1990, p. 53).

References

Fielding, J.A. (1994) Imaging the eye with ultrasound. *Br J Optom Disp*, **2**, 94–102
Retzlaff, J.A. *et al.* (1990) Development of the SRK/T intraocular lens implant power calculation formula. *J Cataract and Ref Surg*, **16**, 333–340
Smith, M.E. *et al.* (1990) In *Noninvasive Diagnostic Techniques in Ophthalmology* (ed. B.R. Masters), Springer, New York, pp. 52–53
Storey, J.K. (1981) The Marton lecture: ultrasound in ophthalmic optics. *Ophthalmic and Physiol Opt*, **1**, 133–158

19 The first three items, A, B and C, do not represent accepted opinion; see Ellis (1986), pp. 14–15 and Harris (1987). For the correct item (D), see Fletcher (1986) in Ellis (1986), pp. 243–244, and Perez-Carpinelli *et al.* (1994).

References

Ellis, D. (ed.) (1986) *Sensory Impairments in Mentally Handicapped People*, Croom Helm, London
Harris, S.R. (1987) In *The Effectiveness of Early Intervention for At-Risk and Handicapped Children* (eds M.J. Guralnick and F.C. Bennett), Academic Press, Orlando, p. 182
Perez-Carpinelli, R. *et al.* (1994) Vision evaluation in subjects with Down's syndrome. *Ophthal Physiol Opt*, **14**, 115–121

20 Lacrimal function tests are needed in several clinical situations, various methods having been proposed. Select from the following statements the one which is correct.

  A The original Schirmer test indicates that tears secretion is normal if 25 mm of the paper strip becomes wet within 9 min

  B A modification of the Schirmer test (S2) involves local conjunctival anaesthesia, the insertion of the paper strip and active irritation of the nasal mucosa for 2 min

  C There has been no satisfactory use of cotton thread as an alternative means of measuring tears secretion

  D The tears film break-up time test is most suited to the assessment of the amount of lacrimal secretion, not being affected by inadequacy of mucus or of lipids in the precorneal tears film

21 Which one of the following statements most correctly refers to the Schiøtz tonometer, which has been described as 'portable, sturdy and relatively inexpensive'?

  A It is an applanation device which involves the use of a silver protein paste

  B It has a moving 'plunger' which can be weighted between 5.5 and 15 g

  C It cannot be used on the sclera in cases where the cornea is too distorted

  D The range of pressures indicated for normal eyes is strongly skewed towards low values

Clinical techniques: Answers

20 The only correct item is B, all the others having misleading elements.

References

Cho, P. (1993) The cotton thread test. *Optom and Vision Sci*, **70**, 804–808
Kurihashi, K. *et al.* (1977) A modified Schirmer test. *J Paediat Ophthalmol*, **14**, 390–397
Lupelli, L. (1986) A review of lacrimal function tests in relation to contact lens practice. *Contact Lens J*, **14** (7/8), 4–18; (9), 3–10; (10), 8–19

21 Item B is the only correct one, since A refers to the Maklakov device. Often, reasonable results without local anaesthetic are obtained using the Schiøtz instrument on the sclera. Most data suggest any skewing of pressures to be towards high, rather than low, values of intraocular pressure.

References

Brown, F.G. and Fletcher, R. (1990) *Glaucoma in Optometric Practice*, Blackwell Scientific, Oxford, pp. 34–37
Draeger, J. and Jessen, K. (1978) In *Glaucoma, Conceptions of a Disease* (eds K. Heilmann and K.T. Richardson), Saunders, Philadelphia, pp. 220–222
Hoskins, D.H. and Kass, M.A. (1989) *Diagnosis and Therapy of the Glaucomas*, Mosby, St Louis, pp. 76–79
Cockburn, D.M. (1991) In *Clinical Procedures in Optometry* (eds J.B. Eskridge *et al.*), Lippincott, Philadelphia, pp. 230–232

22 It is useful to classify (grade) opacities of the crystalline lens. Since some success has been achieved in promoting systems, which of the following suggestions is the best?

A There has been very little interobserver agreement when using slit-lamp grading, so a totally different approach has been promoted

B It is unlikely that there can be much agreement between clinical gradings and gradings made from photographs of nuclear cataracts

C The two sketches shown in Figure 2.3 represent approximately equivalent grades in a system adopted for cortical cataracts

D The lens opacities classification system (LOCS) gradings use slit-lamp photographs with a set of reference photographs which can refer to the intensity of nuclear opacity and the extent of opacity elsewhere in the lens

Fig. 2.3 Two alternative types of crystalline lens opacities.

Clinical techniques: Answers

22 Since the first three items are misleading, it is D which should be selected.

References

Chylack, L.T. *et al.* (1988) Lens opacities classification system. *Arch Ophthalmol*, **106**, 330–334

Douthwaite, W.A. and Hurst, M.A. (1993) *Cataract*, Butterworth-Heinemann, Oxford, pp. 41–43

Hockwin, O. *et al.* (1990) In *Noninvasive Diagnostic Techniques in Ophthalmology* (ed. B.R. Masters), Springer, New York, pp. 281–313

Leske, M.C. *et al.* (1988) Evaluation of a lens opacities classification system. *Arch Ophthalmol*, **106**, 327

Murrill, C.A. *et al.* (1994) *Primary Care of the Cataract Patient*, Appleton & Lange, Norwalk, Connecticut, pp. 18–21

23 A patient with a certain binocular condition has large pupils. He closes his better eye and with his 'bad' eye looks through a 3 mm pinhole in an opaque disc. Looking at a mark × on a sheet of white paper, 50 cm away, while agitating the pinhole in rapid small circular movements, he sees the appearance shown in Figure 2.4. Which of the following suggestions is most appropriate?

A He probably has a small heterotropia with eccentric fixation

B He is observing Haidinger's brushes but without a polarizing filter

C He must have VA better than 6/18, as he is actually observing Maxwell's spot

D A strong afterimage is involved, which is being transferred

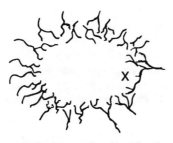

Fig. 2.4 Purkinje 'tree' shadows, using X as fixation point.

24 Measurements of corneal thickness are routinely made with different types of devices, in detailed aftercare of contact lens patients and before and after some types of corneal surgery. In this connection, find the only one of the following statements which is accurate.

A Optical pachometers probably tend to underestimate rather than overestimate corneal thickness

B The technique of specular microscopy cannot be used for measurements of corneal thickness

C A-scan, rather than B-scan, methods of ultrasonography are the basis of ultrasonic pachometry

D There have been insignificant or no differences between corneal thicknesses measured with different types of ultrasonic pachometers

23 While the other three items should each cause recall of some aspect of the investigation of central vision, they are all misleading and inappropriate. It is the Purkinje tree which is being observed, which can often be used to measure the eccentricity and which could be compared to what is seen with the 'good' eye; hence item A is correct. If it is some time since you tried this, observe the normal effect now.

References

Boer, P. and Hofstetter, H.W. (1972) An entopic method for the measurement of eccentric fixation in amblyopia ex anopsia by B. Koppenberg. *Am J Optom Arch Am Acad Optom*, **49**, 417–422

Stidwill, D. (1990) *Orthoptic Assessment and Management*, Blackwell Scientific, Oxford, p. 45

24 Both A and B are the reverse of what is normally understood. As for D, it has been found that there are varied transducers and contact procedures, with different types of power supplies used in different ultrasonic instruments. These appear capable of producing differences in performance, hence the need for careful calibration (see Waring, 1992, pp. 425–429).

Statement C should be chosen (see Waring, 1992, p. 411).

References

Gromacki, S.J. and Barr, J.T. (1994) Central and peripheral corneal thickness in keratoconus and normal patient groups. *Optom and Vision Science*, **71**, 437–441

Grosvenor, T. (1994) In *Contact Lens Practice* (eds M. Ruben and M. Guillon), Chapman and Hall, London, pp. 414–424

Kaufman, H.E. *et al.* (1988) *The Cornea*, Churchill Livingstone, New York, p. 859

Koester, C.J. and Roberts, C.W. (1990) Wide-field specular microscopy. In *Noninvasive Diagnostic Techniques in Ophthalmology* (ed. B.R. Masters), Springer, New York, p. 104

Patel, S. and Stevenson, R.W.W. (1994) Clinical evaluation of a portable ultrasonic and a standard optical pachometer. *Optom and Vision Science*, **71**, 43–46

Stevenson, R.W.W. and Eadie, A.S. (1990) Automated recording and analysis of pachometry data: a technical note. *Contact Lens J*, **17**, 323–326

Waring, G.O. (1992) *Refractive Keratotomy*, Mosby, St Louis

25 Rose Bengal is a somewhat irritant stain used for external
    structures of the eye and the eye region. Which of the following
    statements is least likely to be a correct one?

    A The stain is taken up by living corneal cells but not by dead
       cells
    B The line of Marx, stained along the margin of the lower lid,
       lies behind the orifices of the Meibomian glands
    C In keratoconjunctivitis sicca, this stain is taken up in regions
       of both cornea and conjunctiva
    D The transition of the back of a hard corneal lens may cause
       a stained crescent after the use of this red stain

26 A neutral density (ND) filter test (Ammann, 1921) has some use
    when investigating amblyopia. Which of the following
    statements is the most reliable?

    A Letter acuity is likely to be lower when a case of organic
       amblyopia views an optotype through a 2.5 ND filter but
       strabismic amblyopia would probably show higher letter
       acuity
    B Organic amblyopia (e.g. from a retinal lesion) should be
       suspected in an otherwise normal eye if an ND filter reduces
       visual acuity, even in anisometropic situations
    C An eye with organic amblyopia is likely to suffer a dramatic
       reduction in visual acuity when using a 2.5 ND filter,
       whereas in strabismic amblyopia retinal rod receptors tend
       to maintain the visual acuity. However, in anisometropia the
       rod sensitivity may be impaired
    D Optic neuritis may cause amblyopia, in which case visual
       acuity should actually increase if an ND filter is used

Clinical techniques: Answers

25 Item A is the least likely because it is actually dead cells which Rose Bengal stains, according to most authorities. The last three statements can all be accepted as correct. However, Feenstra *et al.* (1992), in an extended study, showed some possible staining of live cells, a point worth making with some caution.

References
Bartlett, J.D. and Jaanus, S.D. (1989) *Clinical Ocular Pharmacology*, 2nd edn, Butterworths, Boston
Feenstra, A. *et al.* (1992) *Arch Ophthalmol*, **110**, 984–993
Norn, M.S. (1983) *External Eye – Methods of Examination*, 2nd edn, Scriptor, Copenhagen, pp. 60–62
Spalton, D.J. *et al.* (1984) *Atlas of Clinical Ophthalmology*, Churchill Livingstone, Edinburgh, p. 6.11
Terry, J.E. (ed.) (1984) *Ocular Diseases*, Butterworths, Boston, pp. 170, 401 and 593

26 The 'correct' choice is C since all the others tend to be misleading.

References
Ciuffreda, K.J. *et al.* (1991) *Amblyopia. Basic and Clinical Aspects*, Butterworth-Heinemann, Boston, pp. 336–341
Hess, R,.F. and Plant, G.T. (eds) (1986) *Optic Neuritis*, Cambridge UP, Cambridge, pp. 114–118
Mein, J. and Trimble, R. (1991) *Diagnosis and Management of Ocular Motility Disorders*, 2nd edn, Blackwell Scientific, Oxford, p. 60
Newman, N.M. (1991) *Neuro-ophthalmology*, Appleton & Lange, Norwalk, Connecticut, p. 57
Pratt-Johnson, J.A. and Tillson, G. (1994) *Management of Strabismus and Amblyopia*, Thieme, New York, p. 80
Stidwill, D. (1990) *Orthoptic Assessment and Management*, Blackwell Scientific, Oxford, p. 41

27 The selection of letters used for British Standard distance test charts was based on similar legibility and was as follows: D. E, F, H, N, P, R, U, V, Z.

Since it is possible that at least under certain circumstances some of these letters are 'easier' than others for amblyopic subjects, which of the following suggestions is the one which is correct?

A   With visual acuity about 6/18 an amblyope finds the three letters F, R, H much easier to identify than Z, V, U

B   Abnormal monocular fixation by amblyopic eyes tends to produce better visual acuity

C   Amblyopic eyes tend most readily to identify end letters (first/last) on a line of an optotype

D   Crowding, which encourages contours to interact, makes it more accurate to use a standard optotype for amblyopes than for normals

28 Various specifications have been given for optotypes or test charts, such as British Standard (BS 4274: 1968). These may be applied to letters, to 'the illiterate E' and to Landolt rings. Which of the following options is correct?

A   The legibility of selected letters used in charts tends to be slightly better (tending to higher visual acuity) as compared to the legibility of Landolt rings

B   Landolt rings of size 5 $\times$ 5 are likely to indicate a lower visual acuity than when selected 5 $\times$ 4 letters are used in optotypes

C   Non-serif Roman capital letters in the series A, B, C, J, S, W have a greater and more uniform legibility than the series D, E, F, H, N, P when used in optotypes

D   The letters A, H, I, M, O, T, U, V, W, X, Y are those most likely to be used in optotypes, since they are suitable for viewing with or without a mirror

27 The only correct statement is C. Item A is stated in a manner opposite to the accepted comparison of the sets of letters. Items B and D do not represent correct views.

References

Ciuffreda, K.J. *et al.* (1991) *Amblyopia. Basic and Clinical Aspects*, Butterworth-Heinemann, Boston, pp. 320–328

Flom, M.C. (1966) New concepts in visual acuity. *Optom Weekly*, **57**, 63–68

28 While item D contains a partial truth, that range of letters is not widely accepted and used in entirety. Item A is the correct one, since there is a *size correction factor* of approximately 0.95 which should be used to compensate; typical letters in use should be about 15% smaller than rings to produce comparable visual acuity data. In option C the second series, D–P, is extended with R, U, V and Z in BS 4274 (1968). Note the similarity between letters used in Bailey–Lovie distance charts and the BS selection. Note, also, how the Lighthouse (New York) distance chart and Sloan optotypes include S, C and K.

References

Faye, E.F. (1984) *Clinical Low Vision*, 2nd edn, Little, Brown, Boston, p. 28

Grim, W. *et al.* (1994) Correlation of optotypes with the Landolt ring. *Optom and Vision Science*, **71**, 6–13

Lovie-Kitchin, J.E. and Bowman, K.J. (1985) *Senile Macular Degeneration*, Butterworth, Boston, p. 161

29 A patient has partial sight and you wish to determine the magnification needed for reading. The best (reading) spectacle correction is already in place, giving a certain unsatisfactory visual acuity for an habitual reading distance. Here are a number of steps for you to take, each given a number but in random order. Select the optimum order from the four possible orders given later as A to D.

(i) Lend the patient an appliance for home trial
(ii) Increase the near addition and/or decrease the working distance by × (log unit) steps
(iii) Decide what size of words the patient hopes to see
(iv) Test patient's performance with a proposed new addition
(v) Decide on the number of log unit steps between the size found in (iii) and the visual acuity found with the 'normal' addition
(vi) If the improvement in visual acuity is not what you want, go back to the start and try something else

Possibilities:

A (i)→(ii)→(iii)→(iv)→(v)→(vi)
B (ii)→(iii)→(v)→(vi)→(i)→(iv)
C (iii)→(v)→(ii)→(vi)→(iv)→(i)
D (iii)→(v)→(ii)→(iv)→(vi)→(i)

30 Javal's rule in its original form suggests that the spectacle plane astigmatism of an eye equals 1.25 times the astigmatism found with the keratometer, with the addition of $-0.50\,DS \times 90$. The rule has limitations, so which of the following suggestions is most likely to be correct?

A With some exceptions, corrections between $1.00\,DC \times 180$ and $2.00\,DC \times 180$, which are indicated by Javal's rule, are often reasonably close to the subjective astigmatic corrections
B While keratometers are often calibrated for a refractive index of 1.376, the actual corneal refractive index is more like 1.3375
C It is likely that the tilting of the crystalline lens usually introduces into the correct subjective astigmatic error about $1.00\,D$ of 'with-the-rule' astigmatism
D Javal's rule can be applied simply and accurately to cases of oblique astigmatism

29 The optimum sequence is D, which is the most logical one.

References

Faye, E.E. (1984) *Clinical Low Vision*, 2nd edn, Little, Brown, Boston, pp. 50–53

Lovie-Kitchin, J.E. and Bowman, K.J. (1985) *Senile Macular Degeneration*, Butterworth, Boston, p. 95 (this is the best statement of the particular sequence suggested)

Sloan, L.L. and Habel, A. (1956) Reading aids for the partially blind. *Am J Ophthalmol*, **42**, 863–872

Sloan, L.L. (1977) *Reading Aids for the Partially Sighted*, Williams & Wilkins, Baltimore, pp. 79–80

30 Item A is the only correct one. In item B the refractive indices are only correct if transposed. Items C and D are misleading and incorrect.

References

Bennett, A.G. and Rabbetts, R.B. (1989) *Clinical Visual Optics*, 2nd edn, Butterworths, London, pp. 471–472

Elliot, M. *et al.* (1994) Accuracy of Javal's rule in the determination of spectacle astigmatism. *Optom and Vision Sci*, **71**, 23–26

Waring, G.O. (1992) *Refractive Keratotomy*, Mosby, St Louis, p. 62

31 Myopia of 1.50 D in an otherwise normal eye with an average size pupil and reasonably standard (distance) test conditions lowers the unaided vision to some extent. The same amount of astigmatism usually lowers vision to a different extent. Which of the following is most likely to correspond to 1.50 D of myopia?

A   6/36
B   6/18
C   6/24
D   6/60

32 Preferential looking (PL) techniques and the rather simpler acuity card (AC) methods are alternative approaches to the testing of some aspects of infant vision. Which one of the following suggestions is valid?

A   Neither PL nor AC testing can be used until an infant is 24 months old
B   In Dobson's AC procedure the operator knows neither the size nor the location of the grating
C   Newborn infants have never demonstrated PL, in terms of fixation times
D   Psychological 'staircase' methods cannot be applied to PL procedures

33 Tests for stereoscopic acuity can be carried out at different distances, such as 6 metres, or reading distance. There are accepted normal values although these may be modified by test methods. Which *three* of the following items are most likely to be correct?

A   A typical test of stereopsis at 6 m is performed better by orthophoric subjects than by those with intermittent strabismus
B   Near vision stereopsis, evaluated by typical tests, is usually worse than stereopsis measured at 6 m
C   Stereo acuity normally deteriorates with age, so by age 40 years performance is half as good as that which was achieved by the same person at age 18 years
D   Stereo acuity measured by a 'three needle' test at 6 m is likely to be as good as 4 sec of arc, assuming a normal and experienced subject
E   Some subjects, particularly the very young, may take several seconds to appreciate the depth effect presented by clinical stereo tests

Clinical techniques: Answers

31 Item C is correct.

References

Allen, R.J., Fletcher, R. and Still, D.C. (1991) *Eye Examination and Refraction*,
Blackwell Scientific, Oxford, p. 86
Bennett, A.G. and Rabbetts, R.B. (1989) *Clinical Visual Optics*, 2nd edn,
Butterworths, London, p. 112

32 Item B, alone, is valid.

References

Dobson, V. *et al.* (1990) The acuity card procedure: interobserver agreement in
infants with perinatal complications. *Clin Vision Sci*, **6**, 39–48
Dodwell, P.C. *et al.* (1987) In *Handbook of Infant Perception* (II)
(eds P. Salapatek and L. Cohen), Academic Press, Orlando, pp. 7–8
(describes the preferential looking success of Fantz in 1958 with
the newborn)
Lewis, T.L. *et al.* (1993) An evaluation of acuity card procedures. *Clin Vision
Sci*, **8**, 591–602
Thompson, C. (1993) In *Visual Problems in Childhood* (ed. T. Buckingham),
Butterworth-Heinemann, Oxford, p. 172

33 Items A, D and E should be considered to be most likely. Item
B is expressed as the opposite of the usual comparison found.
Most normal subjects do not deteriorate as fast as is suggested
in item C.

References

Bennett, A.G. and Rabbetts, R.B. (1989) *Clinical Visual Optics*, 2nd edn,
Butterworths, London, p. 231
Rosenbloom, A.A. and Morgan, M.W. (eds) (1993) *Vision and Aging*,
Butterworth-Heinemann, Boston, pp. 187–188
Rutstein, R.P. *et al.* (1994) Distance stereopsis in orthophores, heterophores and
intermittent strabismics. *Optom and Vision Sci*, **71**, 415–421

34 Progression of myopia in young patients has been attributed to many possible factors. Some of these have been studied and various approaches to prescribing corrective spectacles have been used. Which two of the following items are most likely to be correct?

A   There is usually relatively little progression of myopia in all children who have been prescribed a full distance correction (over –3.00 D) combined with +2.50 DS addition in bifocal form

B   A longitudinal study of 68 myopic children over a period of up to 9 years showed no definite relationship between changes of height and/or weight and progression of myopia

C   Myopic children (over –3.00 D) with esophoria at 33 cm and prescribed a full distance correction with +2.50 DS addition in bifocal form have a better chance of small progression than those with exophoria at 33 cm

D   When myopia progresses it is usually because an increase in the power of the crystalline lens, or of the cornea, has taken place, without changes in axial length having been involved

35 High myopia presents some special difficulties when using conventional clinical tests. Select from the following items and methods the one most likely to be appropriate in high myopia.

A   Direct ophthalmoscopy is preferable to indirect ophthalmoscopy on account of the larger field of view provided by the direct method

B   Field defects such as concentric contraction and an enlarged blind spot are common and best investigated with contact lens correction

C   Binocular indirect ophthalmoscopy and scleral depression for extreme peripheral examination are unsuitable in such cases

D   Three 10-minute sessions improving flexibility of accommodation should improve distance visual acuity by 3 to 4 'lines' in high myopes

Clinical techniques: Answers

34 Items B and C should be chosen. Certainly there are exceptional cases but the relative merits of the items above are generally agreed as stated.

References

Grosvenor, T. and Scott, R. (1993) Three-year changes in refraction and its components in youth-onset and early adult-onset myopia. *Optom and Vision Sci*, **70**, 677–683

Jensen, H. (1991) Myopic progression in young school children. *Acta Ophthalmologica*, Suppl. 200, **69**, Scriptor, Copenhagen

35 Item B should be chosen as the other items are incorrect.

References

Bell, G.R. (1993) Biomechanical considerations in high myopia: Part III. *J Am Optom Ass*, **64**, 346–351

Koslowe, K.C. *et al.* (1991) Evaluation of accommodative biofeedback training for myopia control. *Optom and Vision Sci*, **68**, 338–343

36 There are limits to the accuracy of refractive procedures and measurements of ametropia and heterophoria. Identify which of the following are the two most likely to represent informed opinion.

A   The standard deviation of measurements of heterophoria is approximately 2 prism dioptres

B   With the same subject, the spherical ametropia measured by different optometrists can be different by up to 0.50 D

C   The physiological tolerance to changes in spherical power, within which no adjustment of accommodation is likely, can be ±0.75 D

D   The perceptual tolerance to changes in spherical power, within which no adjustment of accommodation is likely, can suggest refractive states (including accommodation) between +3.25 D and +5.00 D for an object at 25 cm

37 In slit lamp examination a narrow but variable width, uniformly bright slit must be projected into the ocular tissues. Assuming that the source of light must be a very small coiled filament of tungsten, which of the following arrangements is the best optical system to use? (Rough diagrams of each suggestion should assist the reader.)

A   A white glass diffuser is put between the source and a metal stenopaeic slit. An image of the slit is formed by two positive lenses, one very near the slit and the other nearer the eye

B   An image of the source is formed on a slit in a metal plate, by two positive lenses. An image of the slit is then formed on the eye by a single achromatic lens

C   A positive lens forms an image of the source on a white glass diffuser, from which light immediately passes through a slit. This slit is imaged on the eye by a lens

D   Two positive lenses A and B form an image of the source on a third positive lens. Light passes through a slit which is immediately after lens B while the third lens forms an image of the slit on the eye

Clinical techniques: Answers

36 Items C and D misquote the likely tolerances which exist. Thus items A and B should be chosen as most likely.

References
Allen, R.J., Fletcher, R. and Still, D.C. (1991) *Eye Examination and Refraction*, Blackwell Scientific, Oxford, p. 96
Bannon, R.E. (1977) A new automated subjective optometer. *Am J Optom Physiol Opt*, **54**, 433–438
Hebbard, F.W. (1952) Consistency of clinical data. *Optom Wkly*, **32**, 1269–1273
Morgan, M.W. (1977) The reliability of clinical measurements with special reference to distance heterophoria. *Am J Optom Physiol Opt*, **54**, 433–438

37 Item D is the best system, which is that proposed by Vogt and is virtually the principle of the slide projector. The third lens receives a 'Maxwellian view' of a uniformly illuminated slit; there is the best chance of a bright and uniform slit image. While diffusers have been used in some commerical slit lamps, such diffusers are now chiefly reserved as a temporary cover for the projection lens to give bright widespread diffuse illumination.

References
Berliner, M.L. (1949) *Biomicroscopy of the Eye*, Hoeber, New York
Doggart, J.H. (1948) *Ocular Signs in Slit Lamp Microscopy*, Kimpton, London
Harrison Butler, T. (1927) *An Illustrated Guide to the Slit Lamp*, Oxford University Press, Oxford
Henson, D.B. (1983) *Optometric Instrumentation*, Butterworths, London, p. 122

38 There is at least one way of rating the efficiency of a pseudoisochromatic plate used for colour vision tests, based on the extent to which it classifies subjects into the correct/incorrect categories. Which *two* of the following apply to this approach?

A   Sheard's criterion
B   Sloan–Green criterion
C   Judd's criterion
D   Crooke's criterion

39 During retinoscopy, fixation is sometimes oblique to the axis along which retinoscopy takes place. Suppose that a (monocular) patient looks at a distant object, which is seen to the patient's left of the practitioner who is using a retinoscope with the right eye. The angle between the retinoscopic axis and the patient's line of sight is assumed to be 15 degrees and the patient is emmetropic. Which one of the following possibilities is most likely to be correct?

A   An error in the measured prescription will be introduced which will be too much myopic but it will be a spherical error
B   An error will be introduced which will be both myopic and (obliquely) astigmatic
C   An error will be introduced, both hyperopic and (obliquely) astigmatic
D   Any oblique or radial astigmatism introduced should be over 0.75 D

38 Both B and C are correct. Sheard's criterion is related to heterophoria. Item D is fictional!

Reference

Cline, D., Hofstetter, H.W. and Griffin, J.R. (1989) *Dictionary of Visual Science*, 4th edn, Chilton Trade, Radnor, p. 161

39 Item D is correct, assuming the obliquity suggested in items B and C refers only to meridians significantly near to 45 or 135 degrees Standard Notation. Using a Gullstrand (2) eye, Bennett (1951) calculated that about 1.20 D of 'total radial astigmatism' would be likely with such obliquity between the retinoscopic and visual axes.

References

Bennett, A.G. (1951) Oblique refraction of the schematic eye as in retinoscopy. *Optician*, **120**, 583–588
Millodot, M. and Lamont, A. (1974) Refraction of the periphery of the eye. *J Opt Soc Am*, **64**, 110–111

40 Retinoscopes use either fully silvered mirors with a sight hole for the retinoscopist or a semireflecting mirror which reflects and transmits only part of the incident light. Assume that a patient's retina reflects about 20 per cent of incident light, mostly of long wavelengths. Which of the following suggestions does *not* correctly represent the performance of a retinoscope with a partially reflecting mirror?

A   If the mirror reflects 10 per cent and transmits 90 per cent the patient receives about 10 times as much light as the retinoscopist receives, with which to observe the retinoscopic reflexes

B   If the mirror reflects and transmits 50 per cent the patient receives about 15 times as much light as that which reaches the retinoscopist

C   Increasing the mirror's reflection factor from 40 per cent to 65 per cent sends more light to the patient but reduces the amount of light received by the retinoscopist

D   Increasing reflection from 10 per cent (clear glass) to 40 per cent sends more light to the patient but the retinoscopist receives less light

41 Applanation tonometry uses the principle that the area of corneal flattening produced by a known weight acting on a flat end-plate is directly proportional to the intraocular pressure (IOP). Which of the following is most likely to be correct?

A   A patient must be supine before any form of applanation tonometer can be used with accuracy

B   An applanation tonometer weighing between 6 and 16 g displaces between 15 and 16 mm^3 of intraocular fluid

C   When a corneal diameter of 3.06 mm is applanated with a Goldmann tonometer, the two broken rings which were first observed form a complete, unbroken circle

D   The force on a rigid flat probe applanating the cornea for IOP measurement should flatten both front and back corneal surfaces

40 Statement D is the only incorrect one. With 10 per cent reflection the patient receives about 11 times the light received by the retinoscopist; this would tend to reduce the pupil diameter and would be 'glaring' for the patient. The 40 per cent reflection in item C sends a good amount of light to both persons and is probably optimal. Optometrists should understand the instruments which they use. It is useful to consider and to try an orange filter placed between the retinoscope lamp and the mirror.

Reference

Allen, R.J., Fletcher, R. and Still, D.C. (1991) *Eye Examination and Refraction*, Blackwell Scientific, Oxford, pp. 74–77

41 Item D is correct. The others are incorrect. The tonometer mentioned in item B would displace only about 2.7 mm^3 of fluid. Two half circles should be adjusted, not to form an unbroken circle but so that their inner margins are just touching.

References

Duke-Elder, W.S. (1968) *System of Ophthalmology*, IV, Kimpton, London, pp. 231–233

Perkins, E.S. (1953) A simple applanation tonometer. *Trans Opthalmol Soc*, **LXXIII**, 261–266

Voke, J. (1994) Tonometry – ancient and modern. Part 1. *Br J Optom Disp*, **2**, 271–275

Wolfe, M. (1988) Tonometry. In *Optometry* (eds K. Edwards and R. Llewellyn), Butterworths, London, p. 386

42 The form of visual acuity known as grating acuity, using variations of spatial frequency of a black and white grating, has applications when estimating the visual performance of infants. Variations of the 'preferential looking' method exist which use pictures of familiar objects. Which of the following is most likely to be correct?

A   Using preferential looking stimuli in the form of pictures an infant's visual acuity is likely to be underestimated rather than overestimated, as the stimuli probably represent well-known objects

B   The method of acuity card testing uses gratings presented on either side of the observer's peephole on a suitable grey background, relying on the observer's decision rather than standard psychophysical procedures

C   Dobson's procedure for preferential looking tests enables the operator to know the actual location of each grating which is shown and the actual size of each grating as each is presented

D   STYCAR tests incorporate a highly developed type of preferential looking evaluation, most suitable for children aged between 14 and 36 months of age

43 Lasers of different types have a variety of applications in the investigation of ocular function as well as in treatment of eye conditions. Which one of the following items is the most likely to be incorrect?

A   Using interference patterns formed on the retina with low-power laser radiation, the optics of an eye can be bypassed and an estimate of eventual possible visual acuity can be made before cataract operations

B   A confocal laser scanning ophthalmoscope permits direct measurements of the thickness of nerve fibre layers in the retina; the illumination is through a very small aperture and reflected light is detected through another aperture

C   Argon lasers, with a wavelength of about 500 nm, are absorbed by the ocular media to the extent of approximately 55 per cent

D   Laser treatment of vascular retinopathy usually requires radiation which will be absorbed well by the retinal pigment epithelium

Clinical techniques: Answers

42   Item B is the only correct one. Pictures, with no crowding features, may overestimate visual acuity. Acuity cards, while not a real substitute for preferential looking, probably give reasonably similar results in a shorter time. Dobson's approach gives minimal clues and bias to the operator. The STYCAR series does not involve PL.

References

Dobson, V. *et al.* (1990) The acuity card procedure: interobserver agreement in infants with perinatal complications. *Clin Vision Sci*, **6**, 39–48

Evans, B. (1994) Through the eyes of children. *Optician*, **208**, 26–27

Lewis, T.L. *et al.* (1993) An evaluation of acuity card procedures. *Clin Vision Sci*, **8**, 591–602

Press, L.J. and Moore, B.D. (1993) *Clinical Pediatric Optometry*, Butterworth-Heinemann, Boston, pp. 37–40

43   Item C is incorrect. The absorption is about 5 per cent.

References

Dreher, A.W. and Reiter, K. (1992) Retinal laser ellipsometry: a new method for measuring the retinal nerve fibre layer thickness distribution. *Clin Vision Sci*, **7**, 481–488

Hess, R.F. (1981) In *Clinical Applications of Visual Psychophysics* (eds L.M. Proenza *et al.*), Cambridge University Press, p. 16

Kohner, E. and Hamilton, A.M.P. (1987) In *Clinical Ophthalmology* (ed. S. Miller), Wright, London, p. 238

Miller, D. (ed.) (1987) *Clinical Light Damage to the Eye*, Springer, New York, p. 7

Pitts, D.G. and Kleinstein, R.N. (1993) *Environmental Vision*, Butterworth-Heinemann, Boston, p. 229

Spalton, D.J. *et al.* (1984) *Atlas of Clinical Ophthalmology*, Churchill Livingstone, Edinburgh, p. 1.4

44 The inherited or 'congenital' condition of protanomalous trichromatism is most correctly related to only one of the following items.

  A   It is the most prevalent type of 'colour blindness' found in Europe

  B   The condition can readily be indicated by the D-15 test shown in Figure 2.5, where colour 2 is a blue-green, 11 a red and 13 a reddish-purple

  C   The condition is unlikely to show either difficulty in seeing small dark red lights or an enhanced successive contrast when shown yellow lights after red or green lights

  D   During correct use of a spectral anomaloscope, yellow would be matched with a mixture of more green and less red than is normal

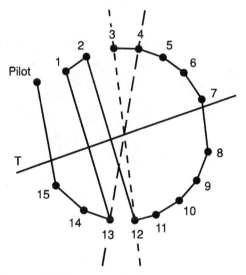

Fig. 2.5   Record of D-15 colour vision test.

44 In Figure 2.5 the confusions correspond with a protan type axis and B is the correct choice. It is deuteranomaly which is most prevalent. Items C and D describe what might well be the reverse of the situation.

References

Birch, J. (1993) *Diagnosis of Defective Colour Vision*, Oxford University Press, p. 31

Boynton, R.M. (1979) *Human Color Vision*, Holt, Rinehart & Winston, New York, p. 378

Fletcher, R. and Voke, J. (1985) *Defective Colour Vision*, Hilger, Bristol, pp. 142, 289, 314 and 325

Kalmus, H. (1965) *Diagnosis and Genetics of Defective Colour Vision*, Pergamon, Oxford, pp. 17 and 42

45 There are several subjective approaches to the study of retinal features, many of these techniques having clinical applications or reinforcing anatomical knowledge. Which one of the following is the correct item?

A Shadows cast by the smallest macular capillaries can be resolved by the neural elements of the retina beneath, which show that the foveal avascular zone is between 0.5 and 0.9 mm in most people

B Observed through a rotating polarizing filter, the movement of the Haidinger brushes (which subtend some 15 degrees) is unchanged by interposing a 'half-wave' plate between the eye and filter

C Maxwell's spot is attributed to the presence of yellow pigment in the region of the macula and is therefore best observed by looking through a yellow filter

D Appropriate stimulation of the retina by dim lights in a dark room reveals the *blue-arcs* phenomenon. By this means it can be shown that fibres from the retinal ganglion cells cross the horizontal raphe

46 Some forms of malingering require careful modifications of standard clinical methods. It is usually best to combine a variety of approaches, for example if blindness is simulated. Which one of the following suggestions is *least likely* to detect the simulation of monocular blindness, which is probably the most common form of simulation?

A The cover test is used, requiring the patient to fixate a distant light. A red filter is placed in front of the 'blind' eye and the patient must name the colour of the light when each eye is uncovered

B A pseudoscope is used, each eye being presented with a stimulus which is apparently being seen by the eye opposite to that which would be most logically expected by the uninitiated

C With the head restrained, the patient is required to read a book while a vertical bar (about 3 cm wide) is held some 12 cm in front of the eyes. Hesitation, or temporary closing of an eye, is noted

D The blind spot of the 'good' eye is plotted on a screen, perhaps 1 to 2 metres distant, but both eyes are uncovered

45 Item A is the only correct one. The others are misleading.

References

Bradley, A. *et al.* (1992) Psychophysical measurement of the size and shape of the human foveal avascular zone. *Ophthal Physiol Opt*, **12**, 18–23

Duke-Elder, W.S. (1968) *System of Ophthalmology*, Kimpton, London, p. 625

Moreland, J.D. (1969) Retinal topography and the blue-arcs phenomenon. *Vision Res*, **9**, 965–976

Sloan, I.I. and Naquin, H.A. (1955) A quantitative test for determining the visibility of the Haidinger brushes: clinical applications. *Am J Ophthalmol*, **40**, 393–406

Voke, J. (1978) Entoptic phenomena and their clinical significance. *Optician*, Sept. 1, 36–39

46 Item A is probably the least likely to be successful.

References

Allen, R.J., Fletcher, R. and Still, D.C. (1991) *Eye Examination and Refraction*, Blackwell Scientific, Oxford, pp. 133 and 208

Duke-Elder, W.S. (1970) *System of Ophthalmology*, V, Kimpton, London, pp. 491–500

Sherman, J. (1994) A revealing new approach to testing. *Br J Optom Disp*, **2**, 401–402

47 A 'reduced' unaccommodated eye is represented by a single surface. A +10.00 DS (thin) lens is placed 15.66 mm in front of this surface (Figure 2.6). There is an object O somewhere in front of the eye and near the eye. An image of O, i, is formed by this lens 184.34 mm behind the ocular surface. The image i acts as a new object, of which the eye forms a sharp image on the retina. One of the following items gives the ocular refractive error, correct to 0.25 D, (also the contact lens correction) needed when the eye is looking at a distant object.

A +10.00 DS
B −6.75 DS
C +5.50 DS
D −5.00 DS

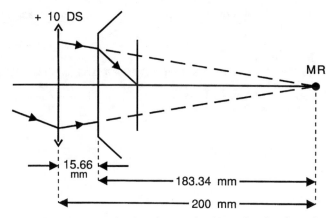

Fig. 2.6 Ray diagram of reduced eye using lens, showing far point.

48 Which of the following describes the method of separation of the right and left eye images in a stereovision test which uses anaglyphs?

A Polarization separates the images
B Colour filters (red masking the red print, and green masking the green print)
C Colour filters (green masking the red print, and red masking the green print)
D A stereoscope is required to separate the images

Clinical techniques: Answers

47 Item C is correct. Since the eye is not accommodating, the position of i must be the far point. The +10.00 DS lens and the eye give a sharp retinal image of the object O, so find the convergence of the light reaching the eye from the lens. There is no need to locate the object because light is known to converge to the image i, reaching the eye with a vergence of 1000/184.34 D = +5.42 D, which is the ocular refractive error and also the required total power of a contact lens correction. A sketch helps.

Reference

Obstfeld, H. (1982) *Optics in Vision*, Ch. 9, Butterworth Scientific, London

48 B is the correct response. These tests differ from bichromatic tests in that they use the colours to give the observer the impression of looking at a picture in monochrome (blackish on whitish).

References

Cline, D., Hofsetter, H.W. and Griffin, J.R. (1989) *Dictionary of Visual Science*, Chilton Radnor, Pennsylvania, p. 28

Rosner, J. and Rosner, J. (1988) *Vision Therapy in a Primary-Care Practice*, Professional Press, New York, p. 66

49 Which one of the following attributes is *not* true of Von Graefe's method of measuring phorias using prism doubling?

A   Good accommodation control

B   May be used for distance and near vision without modification

C   Equally suited to measuring vertical and horizontal deviations, using the same prism for dissociation

D   Requires approximately equal acuity in both eyes

49 C is incorrect. In order to prevent fusion a much larger
horizontal prism is required (for measurement of the vertical
phoria) than vertical. Most refractor heads are fitted with a 6 pd
base up and a 10 pd base in (which may still be inadequate to
prevent fusion). Even so, reasonable results may be obtained for
vertical phoria measurement.

References

Bennett, A.G. and Rabbetts, R.B. (1989) *Clinical Visual Optics*, 2nd edn,
Butterworths, London, p. 205
Borish, I.M. (1970) *Clinical Refraction*, 3rd edn, Professional Press, Chicago,
pp. 810–813

50 A patient complains of sudden onset of double vision when looking to the right. Which two of the following are most likely to be correct?

   A As the more distal image on looking up and to the right is seen by the right eye, the involved muscle is probably the RSR

   B As the more distal image on looking up and to the right is seen by the right eye, the involved muscle is probably the LIO

   C As the deviation is greatest on looking right, with the nearer image seen by the left eye, the RLR is probably involved

   D As the deviation is greatest on looking right, with the nearer image seen by the right eye, the RMR is probably involved

Clinical techniques: Answers

50 A and C are appropriate answers (Figure 2.7).

References
Allen, R.J., Fletcher, R. and Still, D.C. (1991) *Eye Examination and Refraction*, Blackwell Scientific, Oxford, p. 40

Fells, P. (1987) Strabismus. In *Clinical Ophthalmology* (ed. S. Miller), Wright, London, p. 436

Stidwell, D. (1990) *Orthoptic Assessment and Management*, Blackwell Scientific, Oxford, p. 61

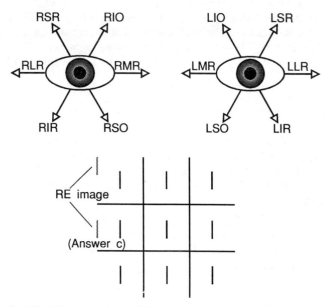

Fig. 2.7 Primary actions of the extraocular muscles are shown at the top, indicating that in situation A the RSR is likely to be involved. The subjective appearances of a 'bar light' stimulus are shown in the lower part, diplopia being evident in the two situations described in the question. The upper left region shows the separation likely for situation A and the middle left region shows that relating to answer C.

51 The cover test may be used to estimate the size of a deviation by judging how far the edge of the limbus moved. As a rough guide which of the following is correct?

A   A movement of 1 mm is the equivalent of 4° or 7 pd
B   A movement of 1 mm is the equivalent of 7° or 4 pd
C   A movement of 1 mm is the equivalent of 1° or 1.3 pd
D   A movement of 1 mm is the equivalent of 1.3° or 1 pd

52 A common error occurs when differentiating between Brown's syndrome (tendon sheath syndrome) and inferior oblique muscle palsy. Which of the following signs is *incompatible* with a diagnosis of Brown's syndrome?

A   Ocular movements which improve with repeated testing
B   V pattern of deviation on testing motility
C   Full development of muscle sequelae
D   Widening of palpebral fissure on adduction

53 The Goldmann tonometer is designed so that when the correct area of applanation is reached, the force flattening the cornea exactly matches the intraocular pressure of the eye, all other forces being balanced. Which of the following statements is correct?

A   The area flattened is equal to $1.75 \, \text{mm}^2$
B   The area flattened is equal to $3.06 \, \text{mm}^2$
C   The area flattened is equal to $7.35 \, \text{mm}^2$
D   The area flattened is equal to $9.36 \, \text{mm}^2$

Clinical techniques: Answers

51 A is correct. Assuming that the limbus is 15 mm from the centre of rotation of the eye then a movement of 1 mm is equivalent to $360/(15 \times \pi)°$, or 3.82°. In order to convert this to prism dioptres, 1 pd is equal to a deviation of 1 cm per metre; see Figure 2.8.

Reference

Bennett, A.G. and Rabbetts, R.B. (1989) *Clinical Visual Optics*, 2nd edn, Butterworths, London, p. 203

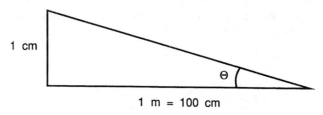

1 cm

Θ

1 m = 100 cm

Fig. 2.8 Trigonometrical features based on an angle of 1 prism dioptre. This is a most important and basic relationship which can be considered in detail as follows: tan Θ 1/100 = 0.01; Θ = 0.573°, i.e. 1 pd = 0.573° or 7 pd = 4°.

52 C is incorrect, being true only of IO palsy in which full development of the ipsilateral SO and contralateral IR sequelae often occurs.

Reference

Mein, J. and Harcourt, B. (1986) *Diagnosis and Management of Ocular Motility Disorders*, Blackwell Scientific, Oxford, p. 301

53 C is the correct area of flattening, being the area of a circle of diameter 3.06 mm. This area of flattening allows the surface tension pulling the tonometer prism onto the eye to compensate for ocular rigidity which resists flattening.

References

Bennett, A.G. and Rabbetts, R.B. (1989) *Clinical Visual Optics*, 2nd edn, Butterworths, London, pp. 369–370

Brown, F. G. and Fletcher, R. (1990) *Glaucoma in Optometric Practice*, Blackwell Scientific, Oxford, pp. 67–69

Davson, H. (1984) *The Eye* (1a), 3rd edn, Academic Press, Orlando, pp. 400–403

54 When setting up a Goldmann tonometer to measure the IOP of a significantly astigmatic patient it is necessary to rotate the prism from its usual horizontally orientated position in order to maintain the correct area of applanation. Which of the following represents the correct amount of rotation?

A 43° from the positive cylinder axis
B Along plus axis of the cylindrical correction
C 43° from the negative cylinder axis
D Along minus axis of the cylindrical correction

55 Which of the following binocular balancing techniques uses a physiological septum?

A Turville infinity balance
B Polarized filters
C Humphriss fogging technique
D Duochrome

Clinical techniques: Answers

54 C is correct. C ensures that the elliptical shape of contact with the cornea has the same area as a circle of 3.06 mm diameter would with a spherical cornea.

References

Bennett, A.G. and Rabbetts, R.B. (1989) *Clinical Visual Optics*, 2nd edn, Butterworths, London, pp. 369–370
Cockburn, D.M. (1991) Tonometry. In *Clinical Procedures in Optometry* (eds J.B. Eskridge, J.F. Amos and J.D. Bartlett), J.B. Lippincott, Philadelphia, p. 222

55 C is correct. The Humphriss fogging technique uses an additional +0.75 or +1.00 DS to blur the image of one eye; this causes the patient to concentrate on the other (in focus) eye while maintaining binocular vision peripherally. As both eyes receive images the septum is, in effect, physiological. The Turville infinity balance uses a physical septum placed on a mirror to ensure that each eye receives a different image. Polarized filters similarly prevent either eye seeing both images while the duochrome is used in monocular balancing techniques.

References

Allen, R.J., Fletcher, R. and Still, D.C. (1991) *Eye Examination and Refraction*, Blackwell Scientific, Oxford, pp. 88 and 98–101
Bennett, A.G. and Rabbetts, R.B. (1989) *Clinical Visual Optics*, 2nd edn, Butterworths, London, pp. 128–132
Wick, B. (1991) Suppression. In *Clinical Procedures in Optometry* (eds J.B. Eskridge, J.F. Amos and J.D. Bartlett), J.B. Lippincott, Philadelphia, p. 703

3 Anatomy & physiology of the eye and vision

1 Parvocellular and magnocellular layers of the lateral geniculate nucleus (LGN) have been associated with different types of visual function. Which of the following alternatives is/are most likely to be correct?

A Two types of retinal ganglion cells are related to their respective layers of the LGN

B More layers of the LGN are concerned with parvocellular function than with magnocellular function

C There is no interaction between the parvocellular and magnocellular systems, even at cortical level

D Parvocellular layers probably contain more colour-opponent units than are found in magnocellular layers

2 Several regions of tissue are normally arranged in order in the human upper eyelid; in fact four planes of tissue have been noted. Starting from the anterior (front) surface and reaching the back surface, which of the following suggestions gives the correct order?

A External skin, subcutaneous tissue, unstriped (Muller's) muscle, areolar tissue, tarsal plate, orbicularis oculi, palpebral conjunctiva

B External skin, areolar tissue, tarsal plate, unstriped (Muller's) muscle, orbicularis oculi, subcutaneous tissue, palpebral conjunctiva

C External skin, subcutaneous tissue, orbicularis oculi, areolar tissue, tarsal plate, unstriped (Muller's) muscle, palpebral conjunctiva

D External skin, areolar tissue, unstriped (Muller's) muscle, orbicularis oculi, tarsal plate, subconjunctival tissue, palpebral conjunctiva

3 Anatomy & physiology of the eye and vision: Answers

1 Items A, B and D have more in their favour than C. It is probably too easy to apply simplifications to the functions involved and there appear to be many opportunities for interactivity between the two systems.

   The parvocellular system is not limited to colour vision although damage to LGN magnocellular layers does not appear to impair much more than perception of motion in the visual field.

References

Davson, H. (1990) *Physiology of the Eye*, Macmillan, London, pp. 504–505
Hagenzieker, M.P. and Van der Heijden, A.H.C. (1993) In *Visual Search 2* (ed. D. Brogan), Taylor & Francis, London, pp. 349–355
Saude, T. (1993) *Ocular Anatomy*, Blackwell Scientific, Oxford, pp. 75–76
Zeki, S. (1993) *A Vision of the Brain*, Blackwell Scientific, Oxford, pp. 186–194

2 Item C is the correct sequence.

References

Duke-Elder, W.S. and Wybar, K.C. (1961) *System of Ophthalmology*, II, Kimpton, London, pp. 507–509
Murray, E.L.J. (1991) The anatomy of the eyelids. *Contact Lens Journal*, **19**(9), 9–14
Saude, T. (1993) *Ocular Anatomy and Physiology*, Blackwell Scientific, Oxford, pp. 89–91
Snell, R.S. and Lemp, M.A. (1989) *Clinical Anatomy of the Eye*, Blackwell Scientific, Oxford, pp. 85–95
Spooner, J.D. (1957) *Ocular Anatomy*, Hatton Press, London, p. 92
Tripathi, B.J. *et al.* (1994) In Ruben, M. and Guillon, M. (eds) *Contact Lens Practice*, Chapman & Hall, London, p. 211

3 The extent of the conjunctival sac is of obvious interest to contact lens practitioners, as it is to wearers who fear loss 'behind the eye'. There are limits to the sac above and below the limbus, nasally as well as temporally and the fornix is located about 5 mm from the orbital margins. Which of the following suggestions most closely represents the extent of the sac from the margins of the normally open eyelids in an adult European male?

A Superiorly 10 mm; nasally zero; inferiorly 6 mm; temporally 20 mm
B Superiorly 5 mm; nasally zero; inferiorly 5 mm; temporally 15 mm
C Superiorly 10 mm; nasally zero; inferiorly 20 mm; temporally 8 mm
D Superiorly 15 mm; nasally zero; inferiorly 10 mm; temporally 6 mm

4 The anatomist Henle described two ocular features of note. Which of the following are the *crypts of Henle*?

A Pits near the root of the iris and/or near the collarette
B Invaginated epithelial sacs, perhaps in the orbital conjunctiva
C Vacuoles in the retina in the perifoveal region
D Spaces in the ciliary epithelium which open into the posterior chamber
E Mobile spaces which move through the endothelium of Schlemm's canal assisting the transport of aqueous humour

5 A structure normally visible with the slit lamp is called a *pigment seam* or *ruff*. Which of the following is the best description of the structure?

A A dark arc or ring of pigment epithelium, related to the borders of the optic disc
B The termination of pigment epithelium at the border of the pupil
C An extent of melanin, trapped when the choroidal fissure closes
D Pigment epithelium which adheres to the anterior lens capsule, but peripheral to the pupil position, following inflammation of the iris

Anatomy & physiology of the eye and vision: Answers

3 Item D is correct. Dimensions are usually given from the limbus or palpebral aperture but experience with scleral lenses reinforces the fact that the sac can be extended to some extent.

References

Duke-Elder, W.S. and Wybar, K.C. (1961) *System of Ophthalmology*, II, Kimpton, London, p. 541
Obrig, T.E. and Salvatori, P.L. (1957) *Contact Lenses*, 3rd edn, Obrig Labs, New York, p. 12
Ruskell, G.L. (1990) The conjunctiva. In *Clinical Contact Lens Practice* (eds W.S. Bennett and B.A. Weissman), Lippincott, Philadelphia, Ch. 3, p. 2

4 Item B is correct. Item A refers to the crypts of Fuchs which lie near the minor iridic circle. Items C, D and E are misleading.

References

Ruskell, G.L. (1990) The conjunctiva. In *Clinical Contact Lens Practice* (eds E.S. Bennett and B.A. Weissman), Lippincott, Philadelphia, Ch. 3, p. 3
Snell, R.S. and Lemp, M.A. (1989) *Clinical Anatomy of the Eye*, Blackwell Scientific, Oxford, p. 32
Spooner, J.D. (1957) *Ocular Anatomy*, Hatton Press, London, p. 27

5 Item B is correct. All the rest are misleading. The pupillary ruff is formed by an extension of the (double) pigmented cells of the iris pigment epithelium which just intrude on to the front of the stroma. It is near the (pupillary) edge of the sphincter muscle, where this muscle curves forwards slightly.

References

Fine, B.S. and Yanoff, M. (1972) *Ocular Histology*, Harper & Row, New York, p. 180
Hogan, M.J. *et al.* (1971) *Histology of the Human Eye*, Saunders, Philadelphia, pp. 211–213
Lowenfeld, I.E. (1993) *The Pupil*, I, Iowa State UP, Ames, p. 26

6 Which of the following statements most accurately describes what happens in the region of the pupil when an isolated very short flash of light is directed at a normal eye?

A   A correspondingly transitory constriction takes place, followed by a dilatation; in fact the *phasic light reflex*
B   Nothing happens until the usual latent period for pupil response, 0.9–1.4 sec
C   The tonic (direct and indirect) light reflex takes place, dilating the pupil for approximately 0.5 sec
D   A state of enhanced pupillary unrest (hippus) is produced, lasting about 30 times the duration of the flash of light

7 Certain structures are found in many parts of the conjunctiva, having the following characteristics: some are elongated cells, most are oval or rounded; their granular cytoplasm contains mitochondria and a Golgi apparatus; possibly they are related to some conjunctival allergies. Which of the following is the best term to apply?

A   Fibroblasts
B   Eosinophils
C   Mast cells
D   Melanocytes

8 Changes in the pupil can take place during a sustained period in a light environment. In this connection, which one of the following statements should you accept as correct?

A   The reflex path controlling the pupil response to light is really an isolated reflex arc
B   The Edinger Westphal part of the oculomotor nucleus stimulates the iris dilator muscle, via the ciliary ganglion
C   In a subject who is startled there is immediate contraction of the pupil dilator muscle but definitely no inhibition of the sphincter muscle
D   Emotional stimuli can impose corticothalamohypothalamic inhibition of the pupil constrictor mechanism

121

Anatomy & physiology of the eye and vision: Answers

6 Item A is correct. Note that latent periods in this connection are normally between 0.2 and 0.5 sec. Hippus, which is usually considered to be pathological, is unaffected by light, yet minor physiological fluctuations can be found as pupillary 'unrest'.

References

Alexandridis, E. (1985) *The Pupil*, Springer, New York, pp. 20–23 and 73
Lowenfeld, I.E. (1993) *The Pupil*, I, Iowa State UP, Ames, pp. 87–88
Lowenstein, O. and Lowenfeld, I.E. (1962) In *The Eye* (ed. H. Davson), 3, Academic Press, London, pp. 249–262

7 Item C is correct.

References

Hogan, M.J. *et al.* (1971) *Histology of the Human Eye*, Saunders, Philadelphia, p. 133
Ruskell, G.L. (1990) In *Clinical Contact Lens Practice* (eds E.S. Bennett and B.A. Weissman), Lippincott, Philadelphia, Ch. 3, p. 7
Tripathi, B.J. *et al.* (1994) In *Contact Lens Practice* (eds M. Ruben and M. Guillon), Chapman & Hall, London, p. 210

8 Item D is correct; the other items are definitely misleading.

References

Hart, W.M. (ed.) (1992) *Adler's Physiology of the Eye*, 9th edn, Mosby, St Louis, p. 420
Lowenstein, O. and Loewenfeld, I.E. (1962) In *The Eye* (ed. H. Davson), 3, pp. 246–247

9 There is a well recognized pupillary reaction to near vision, about which there has been some difference of opinion until fairly recently. Which of the following suggestions do you regard as the single correct one?

  A There is no cortical involvement in the physiology of this reflex

  B Contraction of the ciliary muscle causes blood to fill iris vessels abruptly, contracting the pupil

  C The two (normal) eyes of a subject should have equal near vision reactions but, although they may be as extensive as the light reflex, they may be somewhat slower

  D Squeezing the eyelids very tightly does not produce a near vision constriction but actually produces a dilatation

10 The corneal epithelium forms a smooth covering for the major part of the cornea. Which one of the following composite statements is the most accurate, or even the only correct one?

  A Corneal epithelium, which is normally about three cells thick, is loosely attached to Descemet's membrane

  B Basal cells of the corneal epithelium are normally about 50 microns tall, have no nuclei and do not undergo mitosis

  C The superficial squamous epithelium of the cornea is keratinized, with the cells nearest Bowman's layer being wing-shaped

  D Corneal epithelium, at about 50 microns total thickness, comprises between 8 and 12 per cent of the total corneal thickness

11 In the adult eye there is a layer of neural ectoderm which is not sensory. Which of the following suggestions correctly names this layer?

  A The epithelium running from the iris to the retina

  B The membrane of Bruch, posterior to the ora serrata

  C The anterior cell layer of the crystalline lens, within the capsule

  D Descemet's membrane

9 Item C should be chosen as the correct one, the others being misleading.

References
Alexandridid, E. (1985) *The Pupil*, Springer, New York, pp. 24–25
Hart, W.M. (ed.) (1992) *Adler's Physiology of the Eye*, 9th edn, Mosby, St Louis, p. 418
Lowenfeld, I.E. (1993) *The Pupil*, Iowa State UP, Ames, pp. 295–317

10 Item D is the correct one, the others being incorrect.

References
Fine, B.S. and Yanoff, M. (1972) *Ocular Histology*, Harper & Row, New York, pp. 142–143
Hogan, M.J. *et al.* (1971) *Histology of the Human Eye*, Saunders, Philadelphia, pp. 64–71
Kaufman, H.E. *et al.* (eds) (1988) *The Cornea*, Churchill Livingstone, New York, pp. 5–13

11 Item A is the correct one. Among the others some very strange untruths should be recognized!

References
Barishak, Y.R. (1992) *Embryology of the Eye and its Adnexae*, Karger, Basel, pp. 46–47 and 83
Fine, B.S. and Yanoff, M. (1972) *Ocular Histology*, Harper & Row, New York, pp. 192–199
Hogan, M.J. *et al.* (1971) *Histology of the Human Eye*, Saunders, New York, p. 294

12 A subluxated crystalline lens can be observed with a slit-lamp. Sometimes the zonular fibres appear to be under tension while at the same time the crests of the ciliary processes do not appear to be under tension. Which of the following conclusions about zonular anatomy is most reasonably drawn from such observations?

    A   Zonular fibres are not attached to the ciliary epithelium at all

    B   Most zonular fibres are attached to or merge with the thinnest part of the lens capsule

    C   Zonular fibres do not reach as far as the pars plana of the ciliary body

    D   Most zonular fibres run in the valleys between the ciliary processes

13 A thin, vertical, fibroelastic membrane is attached to a thickened line of periosteum and is associated with the tarsal plates. Which one of the following terms correctly applies?

    A   Tenon's capsule

    B   Orbital septum

    C   Annulus of Zinn

    D   Check ligament(s)

14 The vitreous humour (or *vitreus*) occupies a large part of the eyeball. Which one of the following statements is true?

    A   The major protein of the vitreous, made of polypeptides arranged in a triple helix, is collagen

    B   In the embryo the secondary vitreous has been formed several weeks before the optic vesicle's optic fissure starts to close

    C   It is the primary vitreous in the embryo which makes the largest contribution to the zonule of Zinn

    D   The hyaloid fossa, a space adjacent to the optic disc, is the point of entry for the hyaloid artery into the vitreous

12 Item D is correct.

References

Berliner, M.L. (1949) *Biomicroscopy of the Eye*, Hoeber, New York,
   pp. 1333–1358 (note that this illustrated account is worth seeking out!)
Fine, B.S. and Yanoff, M. (1972) *Ocular Histology*, Harper & Row, New York,
   p. 199
Hogan, M.J. *et al.* (1971) *Histology of the Human Eye*, Saunders, Philadelphia,
   pp. 211–213
Spalton, D.J. *et al.* (1984) *Atlas of Clinical Ophthalmology*, Churchill
   Livingstone, Edinburgh (Fig. 11.16)

13 Item B, otherwise known as septum orbitale, palpebral fascia, or
   even palpebral ligaments, is correct. It is related to the deep
   fascial lining of the palpebral part of the orbicularis muscle.

References

Kaufman, H.E. *et al.* (1992) *Corneal and Refractive Surgery*, Lippincott,
   Philadelphia, p. 264
Rowsey, J.J. (1990) In *Ophthalmic Surgery: Principles and Practice*
   (ed. G.L. Spaeth), Saunders, Philadelphia, p. 204
Saude, T. (1993) *Ocular Anatomy and Physiology*, Blackwell Scientific, Oxford,
   p. 91
Spooner, J.D. (1957) *Ocular Anatomy*, Hatton Press, London, p. 81
Tripathi, R.C. and Tripathi, B.J. (1984) in *The Eye*, 1a, 3rd edn (ed. H. Davson),
   Academic Press, London, p. 87

14 Item A is correct, the others being untrue or misleading.

References

Balazs, E.A. and Denlinger, J.L. (1984) In *The Eye*, 1a, 3rd edn (ed. H. Davson),
   Academic Press, Orlando, pp. 545 and 556–557
Barishak, Y.R. (1992) *Embryology of the Eye and its Adnexae*, Karger, Basel,
   pp. 83 and 105
Davson, H. (1990) *Physiology of the Eye*, 5th edn, Macmillan, London, p. 98
Saude, T. (1993) *Ocular Anatomy and Physiology*, Blackwell Scientific, Oxford,
   p. 40
Sebag, J. (1989) *The Vitreous*, Springer, New York, pp. 8 and 17

15 The normal escape of aqueous humour from the eyeball is a matter of importance and the route through Schlemm's canal has received much attention. Which one of the following statements is *not* true?

   A   The endothelial tissue forming the internal boundary of the canal contains channels which are associated with vacuoles through which aqueous is transported

   B   While the major outflow of aqueous may be via the canal of Schlemm, this route is supplemented by escape through the hyaloid canal and the lamina suprachoroidea

   C   The intrascleral plexus is essentially a series of convoluted arterioles which normally return a high proportion of the aqueous directly into the canal of Schlemm for recycling

   D   There are significant age-related changes in the human trabecular tissues, for example the basal lamina of the fibres thickens, causing a decreased outflow facility

15   Item C is untrue. This plexus, associated with aqueous veins, is
essentially a venous outlet.

References
Brown, F.G. and Fletcher, R. (1990) *Glaucoma in Optometric Practice*,
Blackwell Scientific, Oxford, pp. 202–209
Davson, H. (1990) *Physiology of the Eye*, 5th edn, Macmillan, London,
pp. 40–45
Rohen, J.W. (1978) In *Glaucoma, Conceptions of a Disease* (eds K. Heilmann
and K.T. Richardson), Saunders, Philadelphia, pp. 30–35
Saude, T. (1993) *Ocular Anatomy and Physiology*, Blackwell Scientific, Oxford,
pp. 43–44

16 The blood vessels entering and leaving the eye at the optic disc present a variety of possible normal features when seen with an ophthalmoscope. Figure 3.1 represents at A a common normal arterial variation. Which one of the following suggestions is correct?

A This shows 'situs inversus' associated with tilting of the disc
B The condition is best described as Bergmeister's papilla
C What is shown is a prepapillary arterial loop
D The artery is from the ciliary system and is a cilioretinal artery

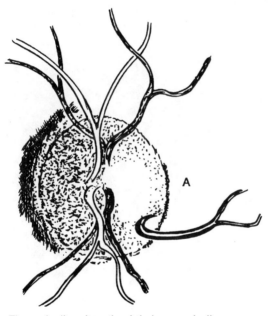

Fig. 3.1 The optic disc viewed ophthalmoscopically.

16 Item D is the correct one. The other terms are valid when applied to the appropriate situations and, if it is not well known, each should be sought in the references.

References

Allen, R.J., Fletcher, R. and Still, D.C. (1991) *Eye Examination and Refraction*, Blackwell Scientific, Oxford, p. 58

Brown, G. and Tassman, W. (1983) *Congenital Anomalies of the Optic Disc*, Grune and Stratton, New York, pp. 31–37; 49–50; 80–87; 171–177

Kritzinger, E.E. and Beaumont, H.M. (1987) *A Colour Atlas of Optic Disc Anomalies*, Wolfe Medical, London, pp. 42–43

Scuderi, G. *et al.* (1987) *Atlas of Clinical Ophthalmoscopy*, Year Book Medical, Chicago, pp. 16–18

Spalton, D.J., Hitchings, R.A. and Hunter, P.A. (1984) *Atlas of Clinical Ophthalmology*, Churchill Livingstone, Edinburgh, p. 14.3

17 In the human crystalline lens, layers of fibres progressively form
various zones. The fibres are elongations of cells contained
within the lens capsule. Which two of the following statements
are correct?

A   Sutures are formed which are visible in the foetal nucleus of
the adult lens in the form of two letters Y, the anterior Y
being inverted when seen from the front of the eye

B   Sutures visible in the adult lens are formed because fibres
starting nearest to the centre in the anterior cortex end
furthest from the posterior pole

C   Secondary lens fibres formed in the 3rd month of gestation
form the inner foetal nucleus; those formed in the 4th month
contribute to the outer foetal nucleus

D   The epithelial cells originally covering the posterior capsule
remain there, extending elongations towards the equator and
towards the front of the lens

17 Items B and C are the correct ones. The other items are
misleading.

References

Barishak, Y.R. (1992) *Embryology of the Eye and its Adnexae*, Karger, Basel,
   pp. 39 and 71
Duke-Elder, W.S. (1961) *System of Ophthalmology*, II, Kimpton, London,
   pp. 322–323
Saude, T. (1993) *Ocular Anatomy and Physiology*, Blackwell Scientific, Oxford,
   pp. 36–38
Snell, R.S. and Lemp, M.A. (1989) *Clinical Anatomy of the Eye*, Blackwell
   Scientific, Oxford, pp. 179–183; 200–201
Spalton, D.J., Hitchings, R.A. and Hunter, P.A. (1984) *Atlas of Clinical
   Ophthalmology*, Churchill Livingstone, Edinburgh, pp. 11.2–11.5

18 Retinal ganglion cells are sometimes responsive to contrast, having receptive fields, parts of which may be excited (+) or inhibited (–) when stimulated by light. Figure 3.2 represents responses of different parts of such a receptive field when a small spot of light is used as a local stimulus. Responses to the periphery (P), to the centre (C) and to both at once (P + C) are shown on the left, with a timed signal S. Which one of the four possible receptive field maps represented on the right corresponds to the pattern of neural responses?

A   on periphery, off centre
B   mixed responses in centre and in periphery
C   off centre, off periphery
D   on centre, off periphery

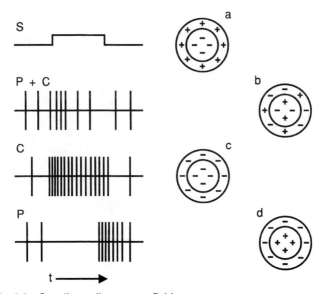

Fig. 3.2   Ganglion cell response fields.

18 Item D is correct. The field shown as D has an 'on' centre which responds to local stimulation and an 'off' periphery which responds only when stimulation of that part of the field ceases. Such retinal ganglion cells function well under conditions of good contrast, such as are provided by small stimuli used clinically in perimeters.

References

Braddick, O. *et al.* (1978) In *Handbook of Sensory Physiology*, VIII (eds R. Held *et al.*), Springer, Berlin, p. 5

Davson, H. (1990) *Physiology of the Eye*, 5th edn, Macmillan, London, pp. 283 and 325

Dowling, J.E. (1987) *The Retina*, Harvard UP, Cambridge, Massachusetts, pp. 33–41

Zeki, S. (1993) *A Vision of the Brain*, Blackwell Scientific, Oxford, pp. 77–78

19 Descriptions of the important central regions of the retina are vital for communication in anatomy, physiology and clinical contexts. Definitions do actually vary according to the context, whether this is histological, functional or clinical. After making a choice as to which one of the following statements is deliberately false, readers would do well to compare the opinions expressed in a number of publications!

A   The macula is approximately 5.8 mm in diameter and subtends about 18.5 degrees when projected on to a wall in front of the eye

B   The foveola is approximately 0.15 mm in diameter and subtends about 1.2 degrees

C   The fovea subtends approximately 5 degrees and is approximately 1.8 mm in diameter

D   The diameter of the macula is approximately 2 mm and this diameter subtends approximately 2 degrees

20 The visual paths extend from the retinal receptors via the optic chiasma to cells in the visual cortex. Which one of the following statements is correct?

A   There are two neurones between the lateral geniculate nucleus (LGN) and the visual cortex, not including cells in the LGN and the cortex

B   Between the receptors and the cortex there are three neurones, not including the receptors and not including the cortical cells

C   Four neurones transmit signals between the retina and the visual cortex, not including the receptors and the cortical cells

D   Between the receptors and the LGN there are three neurones and a single neurone joins the LGN and the cortical cells

19 Item D is the only false statement. One difficulty revolves around a common use of 2 degrees for foveal vision in experimental situations such as colorimetry.

References

Bennett, A.G. and Rabbetts, R.B. (1989) *Clinical Visual Optics*, 2nd edn, Butterworths, London, p. 19
Davson, H. (1990) *Physiology of the Eye*, 5th edn, Macmillan, London, p. 208
Fletcher, R. and Voke, J. (1985) *Defective Colour Vision*, Hilger, Bristol, p. 14
Saude, T. (1993) *Ocular Anatomy and Physiology*, Blackwell Scientific, Oxford, p. 55
Snell, R.S. and Lemp, M.A. (1989) *Clinical Anatomy of the Eye*, Blackwell Scientific, Boston, pp. 169–196
Yanoff, M. and Fine, B.S. (1989) *Ocular Pathology*, Lippincott, Philadelphia, p. 382

20 Item B is the only correct one.

References

Davson, H. (1990) *Physiology of the Eye*, 5th edn, Macmillan, London, p. 207
Fletcher, R. and Voke, J. (1985) *Defective Colour Vision*, Hilger, Bristol, pp. 12–36
Saude, T. (1993) *Ocular Anatomy and Physiology*, Blackwell Scientific, Oxford, pp. 54–81

21 The dioptric scales shown in Figure 3.3 show accommodative responses to a typical series of stimuli to accommodation. Readers must first decide which scale applies to each feature; for example, does the abscissa (with even numbers) refer to responses or to stimuli? The line W shows the theoretical one-to-one matched relationship between stimulus and response. Three curves X, Y and Z indicate accommodative responses for three different subjects. Which *two* of the following statements are most likely to be correct?

A   A normal subject of about 40 years of age is represented by curve X, while line Y applies to some of the responses for a child of a few weeks of age

B   Responses of an amblyopic eye of a subject are shown by curve Z, while curve Y represents those of the dominant and normal eye of the same subject

C   A normal child about 7 years old responds as indicated by curve Z and a normal 11-year-old child is likely to produce curve X

D   The responses of a normal 3-month-old baby might reasonably be shown by curve Z, with curve X representing responses of a normal 42-year-old adult

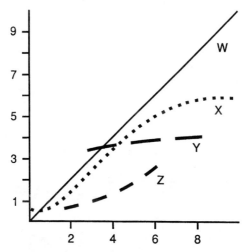

Fig. 3.3 Accommodative responses, stimuli and responses being shown with dioptric scales but without identification as to which is which.

21 Both A and D are likely; the other statements are very misleading and incorrect. The abscissa with the horizontal scale of even numbers in dioptres refers to stimuli and the ordinate with odd numbers indicates dioptres of response. The mismatch between W and X, after stimuli of about 1 D, indicates what is often called 'accommodative lag'. The upper end of curve X shows that the amplitude of accommodation has been reached at about 6 D.

References

Aslin, R.N. (1987) In *Handbook of Infant Perception* (eds P. Salapatek and L. Cohen), I, Academic Press, Orlando, pp. 47–49

Bennett, A.G. and Rabbetts, R.B. (1989) *Clinical Visual Optics*, 2nd edn, pp. 140 and 194

Rosenfield, M. *et al.* (1993) Tonic accommodation: a review. 1. Basic aspects. *Ophthal Physiol Opt*, **13**, 266–284

Ward, P.A. (1985) A brief overview of accommodation. *Optometry Today*, **25**, 725–730

22 Various types of accommodative function have been described and investigated, with considerable acceptance of terms which help to identify the processes involved. Which of the following items is most likely to be correct?

A   Young subjects usually reduce their resting position accommodation by about 0.75 D after some minutes in the dark

B   When all normal stimuli are operational the accommodative mechanism is said to be in *open loop* mode

C   A monocular subject with low visual acuity probably tends to accommodate excessively as a response to a poor retinal image

D   Tonic accommodation is found in *open loop* situations in which there is neither response to retinal image blur nor active convergence

23 There are some differences in anatomical structure between the upper and lower lids and some differences between Oriental and Western eyelids. Such differences may well be important factors in contact lens practice. Which of the following statements is most likely to be correct?

A   The Western upper eyelid has a greater extension of preaponeurotic fat which comes closer to the eyelid margin, producing a lid which looks thicker than the typical Oriental eyelid

B   The upper eyelid, at least in typical Europeans, probably has a squarer shape at the margin, relative to the rounded margin more often found in the middle of the lower lid

C   The Oriental upper lid has a characteristic eyelid crease, usually near the level of the border of the superior tarsal plate, which is less pronounced in the Western upper lid

D   The corrugator supercilii muscle tends to pull the lower lid downwards and away from the nose; as this tendency is greater in Orientals it causes the characteristic slanted palpebral aperture

22 Item D should be selected. Tonic accommodation, lacking any stimuli, is related to the state of innervation of the ciliary muscle; it is very difficult to produce conditions which are free of stimuli, even those related to a sense of nearness of an unseen object.

References

Ciuffreda, K.J., Levi, D.M. and Selenow, A. (1991) *Amblyopia. Basic and Clinical Aspects*, Butterworth-Heinemann, Boston, pp. 261–263

Davson, H. (1990) *Physiology of the Eye*, 5th edn, Macmillan, London, p. 778

Rosenfield, M. *et al.* (1993) Tonic accommodation: a review. I. Basic aspects. *Ophthal Physiol Opt*, **13**, 266–284

23 Item B is most likely to be correct. All the other suggestions are misleading.

It is the relatively less well developed eyelid crease which tends to produce the Oriental slanted eye.

References

Doxanas, M.T. and Anderson, R. (1984) Oriental eyelids: an anatomic study. *Arch Ophthalmol*, **102**, 1232

Murray, E.L.J. (1991) The anatomy of the eyelids. *Contact Lens J*, **19**, (9) 9–16; (10) 17–27

Shanks, K.R. (1965) The shape of the margin of the upper eyelid, related to corneal lenses. *Br J Physiol Opt*, **XXII**, 71–83

24 An early retinal photopigment known as *visual purple* (rhodopsin) is associated with the rod receptors. Which two of the following statements are correct ones and which are incorrect?

   A   Rhodopsin is a chromoprotein which is synthesized at the endoplasmic reticulum and transported to the inner segment of the rod

   B   During the breakdown cycle of rhodopsin, following exposure to light, the meta-rhodopsin stage is earlier than the lumi-rhodopsin stage

   C   When light energy is absorbed by rhodopsin, the structure of the opsin alters in several stages which involves a detachment of retinene

   D   In order to regenerate rhodopsin, several conditions are necessary, chiefly enough vitamin B12 (retinal) and a physical separation between the rods and the pigment epithelium

25 The optic disc, through which retinal fibres leave the eye to join the optic nerve, can be observed with the ophthalmoscope to have several familiar features in most normal emmetropic eyes. Which of the following is most likely to be correct?

   A   Most discs are elliptical in appearance, the long axis usually being approximately horizontal, on account of the common presence of with-the-rule astigmatism

   B   Most discs are circular in appearance, being anatomically elliptical with the long axis horizontal but being magnified more in the vertical direction by with-the-rule astigmatism

   C   Most discs appear to be elliptical with the long axis approximately vertical, usually about 10% longer than the horizontal axis

   D   Most discs appear to be elliptical, long axis horizontal and usually about 30% longer than the short axis, with the long axis most often skewed about 30% nasally

24 Items A and C are correct and the others are incorrect.

References

Arden, G.B. (1976) In *The Eye*, 2A, 2nd edn (ed. H. Davson), Academic Press, New York, p. 242

Davson, H. (1990) *Physiology of the Eye*, 5th edn, Macmillan, London, pp. 232–252

Dowling, J.E. (1987) *The Retina*, Harvard UP, Cambridge, Massachusetts, pp. 197–207

Saude, T. (1993) *Ocular Anatomy and Physiology*, Blackwell Scientific, Oxford, pp. 68–69

Weale, R.A. (1982) *Focus on Vision*, Hodder & Stoughton, London, pp. 24–29

25 Item C is correct. There is usually some contribution to an unequal magnification from with-the-rule astigmatism.

References

Hitchings, R.A. (1987) In *Clinical Ophthalmology* (ed. S. Millar), Wright, London, p. 308

Kritzinger, E.E. and Beaumont, H.M. (1987) *Optic Disc Abnormalities*, Wolf Medical, London, p. 12

Williams, T.D. (1978) Congenital malformations of the optic-nerve head. *Am J. Optom Physiol Optics*, **55**, 706–718

Williams, T.D. (1987) Elliptical features of the human optic nerve head. *Am J Optom Physiol Optics*, **64**, 172–178

26 Visual acuity of whatever type is related to the mosaic of receptors on which a retinal image falls. Identify the only one of the following items which is correct.

A Bipolar cells described as midget are those which are most likely to be involved with activity of a single cone

B Vernier acuity is achieved by using four vertical rows of receptors; the two central rows are stimulated less and respond less than the other rows

C Vernier acuity, being a 'hyperacuity' which is better than conventional visual acuity, is really a matter of spatial localization

D Normal variations of ability to resolve patterns include better resolution when gratings are at 45 degrees to the vertical, than when gratings are vertical

27 The extraocular muscles (EOM) have certain distinctive features which distinguish them from other muscles. Which *two* of the following statements are correct?

A The felder fibres in the EOM are considered to have relatively slow and tonic types of activity

B The oculomotor or third cranial nerve controls all but one of the six EOM

C The fibrille fibres in the EOM operate in conjunction with terminations resembling small bunches of grapes

D Tonic activity can be recorded using suitable electrodes which are inserted into one of the EOM and connected to appropriate apparatus

28 The monocular field of vision is measured with a perimeter. There are individual variations and differences of opinion as to normal limits of the field. There is some relationship to the meridional limits of the ora serrata. Which of the following would you accept as being the most representative of normality?

A 45° up; 45° down; 45° nasally; 90–95° temporally

B 75° up; 45° down; 45° nasally; 90–95° temporally

C 50–55° up; 30–40° down; 60–70° nasally; 95–100° temporally

D 60–65° up; 70–75° down; 55–60° nasally; 95–100° temporally

26   Items A and C should be chosen. The others are misleading.

References
Bennett, A.G. and Rabbetts, R.B. (1989) *Clinical Visual Optics*, 2nd edn, Butterworths, London, pp. 31–32

Blakemore, C. (1978) In *Handbook of Sensory Physiology*, VIII (eds R. Held *et al.*), Springer, Berlin, p. 411

Davson, H. (1990) *Physiology of the Eye*, 5th edn, Macmillan, London, pp. 375–378

De Valois, R.L. and De Valois, K.K. *Spatial Vision*, Oxford University Press, Oxford, p. 248

Westheimer, G. (1979) The spatial sense of the eye. *Invest Ophthalmol Vis Sci*, **18**, 893–912

27   Items A and D should be chosen. The others are misleading.

References
Alpern, M. (1962) In *The Eye*, 3 (ed. H. Davson), *Muscular Mechanisms*, Academic Press, New York, pp. 156–157

Davson, H. (1990) *Physiology of the Eye*, Macmillan, London, pp. 668–671

Saude, T. (1993) *Ocular Anatomy and Physiology*, Blackwell Scientific, Oxford, p. 118

Snell, R.S. and Lemp, M.A. (1989) *Clinical Anatomy of the Eye*, Blackwell Scientific, Boston, pp. 217–228

28   Item D corresponds most closely to the consensus of opinion. This assumes that stimuli and conditions are suitable for the determination of the extreme limits of the field, with a stationary eye.

References
Bennett, A.G. and Rabbetts, R.B. (1989) *Clinical Visual Optics*, 2nd edn, Butterworths, London, p. 179

Giles, G.H. (1960) *The Practice of Refraction*, Hammond, London, p. 372

McClure, E. (1988) In *Optometry* (eds K. Edwards and R. Llewellyn), Butterworths, London, p. 355

Spalton, D.J. *et al.* (1984) *Atlas of Clinical Ophthalmology*, Churchill Livingstone, Edinburgh, p. 1.8

29 The actions of the four extraocular muscles known as recti are affected by the positions at which they are inserted on the eyeball. During some operations for squint (strabismus), these actions are altered by changes in the positions of the insertions. Which one of the following statements is correct for an average eye, before surgery?

A   The superior rectus is inserted nearer to the limbus than the inferior rectus

B   The insertion of the lateral rectus is nearer to the limbus than that of the medial rectus

C   While the medial rectus is inserted 5–6 mm from the limbus, the lateral rectus is inserted about 1–2 mm further from the limbus

D   The superior rectus is inserted about 5 mm from the limbus and the lateral rectus is inserted much nearer than 5 mm from the limbus

30 Figure 3.4 shows five different representations of a vertebrate rod retinal receptor. In each the outer segment, roughly half to one third of the length of the receptor, is drawn in a different way. The orientation of the drawings is not the one usually found in textbooks. Which of the drawings most closely resembles the classical description?

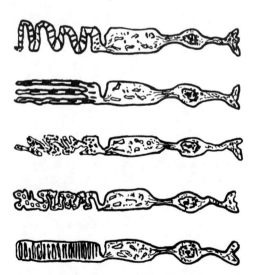

Fig. 3.4 Retinal receptors represented in different ways; four are obviously incorrect sketches.

Anatomy & physiology of the eye and vision: Answers

29 Item C is the only correct one.

References

Davson, H. (1990) *Physiology of the Eye*, Macmillan, London, p. 647
Duke-Elder, W.S. (1961) *System of Ophthalmology*, II, Kimpton, London, p. 426
Saude, T. (1993) *Ocular Anatomy and Physiology*, Blackwell Scientific, Oxford, p. 109
Spalton, D.J. *et al.* (1984) *Atlas of Clinical Ophthalmology*, Churchill Livingstone, Edinburgh, p. 18.9

30 The lowest of the drawings should be chosen. The dark bands across the width of the outer segment indicate the piled discs of photopigment which are formed near the connection with the inner segment.

References

Davson, H. (1990) *Physiology of the Eye*, 5th edn, Macmillan, London, p. 207
Duke-Elder, W.S. (1961) *System of Ophthalmology*, II, Kimpton, London, p. 240
Snell, R.S. and Lemp, M.A. (1989) *Clinical Anatomy of the Eye,* Blackwell Scientific, Boston, p. 163
Weale, R.A. (1982) *Focus on Vision*, Hodder & Stoughton, London, p. 24

31 The lateral walls of the adult orbit each make an angle of about 45 degrees with the sagittal plane and within the orbit the extraocular muscles lie at certain angles to the orbital walls. Various actions of the extraocular muscles depend on the angles at which the eye is pulled during different positions of the visual axes. Which one of the following items is most likely to be correct?

A   When the eyes are in the primary position for distance vision the right and left superior recti each lie at 45 degrees to the medial walls of the two orbits

B   When the two eyes converge maximally all the recti tend to produce an ex cyclo version of the eyes, by rotating the insertions of the superior recti towards each other and towards the sagittal plane

C   During convergence the right superior oblique muscle lies at the same angle to the inferior rectus as it does when the right eye looks as far as possible to the temporal side

D   During convergence the superior recti tend to produce in cyclo rotation of the eyeballs, an action which tends to be compensated by the actions of the inferior recti

32 The ophthalmic artery leaves the internal carotid artery and enters the orbit to supply ocular and nearby tissues. Which of the following is most likely to be accurate?

A   Within the optic canal the ophthalmic artery lies above the optic nerve and is outside the dura mater which covers the nerve

B   The central retinal artery enters the optic nerve before the ophthalmic artery changes its position relative to the optic nerve

C   There are no tributaries of the ophthalmic artery which might supply structures such as sinuses, outside the orbit

D   Ethmoidal arteries, from the ophthalmic artery, and the supraorbital artery enter some sinuses which are close to the orbit

Anatomy & physiology of the eye and vision: Answers

31 Item D should be chosen.

References
Alpern, M. (1962) In *The Eye*, 3, *Muscular Movements* (ed. H. Davson),
Academic Press, New York, pp. 34–40
Saude, T. (1993) *Ocular Anatomy and Physiology*, Blackwell Scientific, Oxford,
pp. 108–117
Solomons, H. (1978) *Binocular Vision*, Heinemann Medical, London, pp. 73–91

32 Item D should be chosen. The ophthalmic artery lies beneath the
nerve within the canal and for some distance within the orbit.
The ophthalmic artery may cross under or over the optic nerve.

References
Barishak, Y.R. (1992) *Embryology of the Eye and its Adnexae*, Karger, Basel,
p. 21
Hayren, S.S. (1976) The ophthalmic artery. In *Vision and Circulation*
(ed. J.S. Cant), Kimpton, London, pp. 171–179
Saude, T. (1963) *Ocular Anatomy and Physiology*, Blackwell Scientific, Oxford,
pp. 128–130
Spalton, D.J., Hitchings, R.A. and Hunter, P.A. (1984) *Atlas of Clinical
Ophthalmology*, Churchill Livingstone, Edinburgh, p. 20.3

33 Pupil size influences several visual functions and their variations during everyday life or during clinical tests. Which one of the following is least likely to be true?

   A   A large, normal pupil is probably associated with poor visual acuity since resolution of objects is adversely affected

   B   A person 60 years old probably has less than half the level of retinal illuminance enjoyed by a 20-year-old, while a 40-year-old should have more than half

   C   People with dark irides living in Africa tend to have smaller pupils than people with light irides living in Belgium

   D   Human pupils can be found with diameters which range from 1.3 mm to over 9 mm

34 A comparison of the concentrations of several substances in the blood and in the aqueous humour reveals some differences. Therefore the term *blood–aqueous barrier* is a convenient one. In this connection, which of the following suggestions is most likely to be correct?

   A   The ciliary epithelium and the capillaries in the ciliary processes together form a complete barrier to the passage of both proteins and non-colloids into the aqueous

   B   While the non-pigmented cells of the ciliary epithelium form part of the blood–aqueous barrier, the endothelial cells of the iris capillaries do not

   C   A flow of aqueous into the ciliary muscle can be considered to be a functional part of the blood–aqueous barrier

   D   Aqueous production is no longer considered to involve secretion; it is actually the result of a simple filtration

33 Item A should be chosen as the least likely statement. Pupils are usually larger during youth, when contrast sensitivity is high and visual acuity has not declined greatly.

References

Lowenstein, O. and Lowenfeld, I.E. (1962) In *The Eye*, 3 (ed. H. Davson), Academic Press, New York, p. 321

Rosenbloom, A.A. and Morgan, M.W. (eds) (1993) *Vision and Aging*, 2nd edn, Butterworth-Heinemann, Boston, pp. 188–191

Weale, R.A. (1963) *The Aging Eye*, Lewis, London, pp. 56 and 144–150

Weale, R.A. (1982) *A Biography of the Eye*, Lewis, London, pp. 276, 279 and 298

34 Item C is a reasonable choice, taking the anatomical parts of the barrier to involve both the non-pigmented cells of the ciliary epithelium and the endothelial cells of capillaries in the iris.

References

Bill, A. (1976) In *Vision and Circulation* (ed. S.S. Hayreh), Kimpton, London (Section on tissue fluid dynamics in the eye)

Cole, D.F. (1984) In *The Eye*, 1a, 3rd edn (ed. H. Davson), Academic Press, Orlando, pp. 303–308

Davson, H. (1990) *Physiology of the Eye*, 5th edn, Macmillan, London, pp. 22–24

35 The *photochromatic interval* is a term used when referring to the ratio of the colour threshold to the threshold for the perception of light. These have sometimes been called the 'specific threshold for colour' and the 'absolute threshold'. Rod and/or cone functions may be involved.

Identify among the following suggestions the one which is correct.

A The photochromic interval is often smallest at the red end of the spectrum
B The density of rods in the human retina is maximal at 2 degrees from the foveola
C At high luminances the relative luminous efficiency of an equal energy spectrum is maximal at wavelength 505 nm
D Visual purple (rhodopsin) absorbs light of wavelength 585 nm or more and therefore has a greater photosensitivity to such light than applies to light of wavelength 505 nm

36 Several observations from visual experiments have formed the bases for various 'laws'. Which of the following laws is most closely related to the phenomenon of flicker, rather than to the absolute visual threshold?

A The Talbot–Plateau law
B Bloch's law
C Piper's law
D Ricco's law

35 Item A is correct.

References

Le Grand, Y. (1968) *Light, Colour and Vision*, 2nd edn, Chapman & Hall, London, pp. 109–112 and 258–259

Saude, T. (1993) *Ocular Anatomy and Physiology*, Blackwell Scientific, Oxford, p. 67

36 Item A is correct. Talbot and Plateau each in 1834 noted that the percept obtained at and over the critical frequency of flicker is that of a constant luminance – the mean value of the luminance(s) being presented over several seconds.

References

Boynton, R.M. (1979) *Human Color Vision*, Holt, Reinhart & Winston, New York, p. 302

Davson, H. (1990) *Physiology of the Eye*, 5th edn, Macmillan, London, p. 362

Le Grand, Y. (1968) *Light, Colour and Vision*, 2nd edn, Chapman & Hall, London, pp. 306–307

37 A certain experiment to determine the critical frequency of flicker (CFF) can use standardized conditions for fixation and stimulus size, starting with intermittent stimuli of white light of a fairly high luminance. Which of the following is most likely to be correct?

   A The sensation of flicker is removed at a certain frequency and then the frequency can be increased slightly, when flicker will return

   B Flicker ceases at a certain frequency, after which the frequency is reduced until flicker is just perceived. Then the luminance is reduced by 50 per cent and the flicker disappears

   C Flicker ceases at a certain frequency, the CFF, after which the frequency is reduced until flicker is just perceived. Then the luminance is increased by 50 per cent and the flicker disappears, unless the frequency is reduced

   D Flicker ceases at the CFF. The luminance is increased, but by decreasing the frequency and increasing the size of the retinal image the absence of flicker can be maintained

38 Various changes take place in retinal function and the resulting sensations as luminance changes from photopic to scotopic levels, through mesopic vision. Which of the following suggestions is the correct one?

   A The Purkinje effect is related to the observation that red and blue objects may appear equally bright in strong daylight but the red object would appear brighter at early dawn

   B The Purkinje effect is not easily observed if the objects which are being observed for relative brightness subtend about 0.75 degrees and are observed with foveal fixation

   C Photopic vision is concerned when an object subtends about 30 degrees, has a luminance of about $0.001 \, cd/m^2$ and is seen within a surround of lower luminance

   D The critical frequency of flicker generally decreases as retinal illuminance increases, assuming that white stimuli are used

37 Item B is correct.

References
Boynton, R.M. (1979) *Human Color Vision*, Holt, Reinhart & Winston, New York, p. 301
Davson, H. (1990) *Physiology of the Eye*, 5th edn, Macmillan, London, pp. 362–363
Le Grand, Y. (1968) *Light, Colour and Vision*, 2nd edn, Chapman & Hall, London, pp. 306–310

38 Item B is correct.

References
Boynton, R.M. (1979) *Human Color Vision*, Holt, Reinhart & Winston, New York, p. 114
Hartridge, H. (1950) *Recent Advances in the Physiology of Vision*, Churchill, London, pp. 35–44
Le Grand, Y. (1968) *Light, Colour and Vision*, 2nd edn, Chapman & Hall, London, pp. 122–123

39 Movements of the eyelids, often associated with eye movements, are important aspects of ocular protection and general well-being. The nerves involved are important during normal function and during abnormal situations. Which *two* of the following items are correct and which two are incorrect?

A The efferent neural path for eyelid closing by the orbicularis and accessory frontalis muscles goes through the zygomatic branches of the oculomotor (III) nerve

B During bilateral actual or attempted closure of the eyelids, there is usually a vertical and downward movement of the eyes, known as Bell's phenomenon

C Reflex blinking occupies about 0.25 seconds, perhaps 7 to 12 times each minute and the rate may almost double during the first few hours of hard corneal lens wearing

D During most acts of binocular blinking the EOM contract sufficiently to pull the eyeballs backwards rather more than 1 mm

40 Most theories of accommodation have been based on observations on living eyes or on anatomical studies. Which one of the following is most likely to be correct?

A When the zonular connections are cut in a fresh eye, between the ciliary processes and the crystalline lens, the lens assumes an unaccommodated and less positive form

B During accommodation there is a slight increase in the depth of the anterior chamber, between the anterior pole of the lens and the back of the cornea

C If a drug or electrical stimulation causes contraction of the ciliary muscle, the zonule increases its tension on the lens, which relaxes any accommodation

D Presbyopia is developed more by alterations in the lens and its capsule than by alterations in the ciliary body and ciliary muscle

Anatomy & physiology of the eye and vision: Answers

39 Items C and D are correct, the others being incorrect. In relation to A, it is the VII nerve which is involved, not the oculomotor nerve. Bell's phenomenon, while not an invariable action, is most likely to involve an upward movement of the globes, which tends to perform a protective function when foreign bodies threaten the eye, as in explosions.

References

Cline, D., Hofstetter, H.W. and Griffin, J.R. (1989) *Dictionary of Visual Science*, 4th edn, Chilton Trade, Radnor, p. 520

Lawson, R.W. (1950) Blinking and sleep. *Nature*, **165**, 81–82

McEwan, W.K. (1962) Secretion of tears and blinking. In *The Eye*, 3 (ed. H. Davson), Academic Press, New York, pp. 290–301

Murray, E.L.J. (1991) The anatomy of the eyelids. *Contact Lens J*, **19**, 9–16

Riggs, L.A. *et al.* (1987) Blink related eye movements. *Invest Ophthalmol Vis Sci*, **28**, 334–340

40 Item D should be chosen, all the others being regarded as untrue.

References

Fincham, E.F. (1937) The mechanism of accommodation. *Br J Ophthalmol*, **8** (Suppl.)

Fisher, R.F. (1973) Presbyopia and the changes with age in the human crystalline lens. *J Physiol*, **228**, 765–779

Stark, I. (1987) Presbyopia in light of accommodation. In *Presbyopia* (eds L. Stark and G. Obrecht), Professional Press, New York, pp. 264–274

41 A normal young emmetrope with plenty of accommodation responds to different stimuli to accommodation in different ways. The conditions and features of the stimuli are important. Which one of the following proposals is most likely to be correct?

    A The spatial frequency of the detail in targets such as small near letters is lowered by optical blurring up to 2 D. Then the accommodative response will have a bias to excessive amounts of accommodation

    B The luminance of small near letter targets is progressively lowered, in which case the accommodative response to the stimuli tends to increase

    C Accommodation usually seeks a resting level in which accommodation is higher than its minimum value

    D Given a large range of stimuli such as sinusoidal gratings of different spatial frequencies, accommodation is not affected by the frequency changes

42 The ciliary ganglion is important because it relays and/or transmits various neural commands to or from structures inside the eyeball. Which two of the following statements are correct?

    A The long ciliary nerves leave the ciliary ganglion bearing both sympathetic and parasympathetic fibres

    B Sympathetic fibres enter the ciliary ganglion by its short root and leave by its motor root

    C Sympathetic fibres, which enter the ciliary ganglion as preganglionic fibres, synapse within this ganglion and leave it as postganglionic fibres

    D Motor fibres enter the ciliary ganglion as preganglionic fibres, synapse within it and leave as postganglionic fibres associated with pupil constriction

Anatomy & physiology of the eye and vision: Answers

41 Item C is correct, as shown by the phenomenon of 'night' (empty field) myopia, which must be considered when prescribing refractive corrections. The other items tend to express the opposite of what might be expected.

References

Charman, W.N. and Tucker, J. (1977) Dependence of accommodation response on the spatial frequency of the observed object. *Vision Res*, **17**, 129–139
Green, D.G. and Campbell, F.W. (1965) Effect of focus on the visual response to a sinusoidally modulated spatial stimulus. *J Opt Soc Am*, **55**, 1154–1157
Heath, G.G. (1956) The influence of visual acuity on accommodative responses of the eye. *Am J Optom*, **33**, 513–524
Nadell, M.C. and Knoll, H.A. (1956) The effect of luminance, target configuration and lenses upon the refractive state of the eye. I and II. *Am J Optom*, **33**, 24–42 and 86–95

42 Items A and D are correct, the others being incorrect distracting suggestions.

References

Davson, H. (199?) *Physiology of the Eye*, 5th edn, Macmillan, London, p. 776
Lowenstein, O. and Lowenfeld, I.E. (1962) In *The Eye*, 3 (ed. H. Davson), Academic Press, New York, p. 248
Ruskell, G.L. and Griffiths, T. (1979) Peripheral nerve pathway to the ciliary muscle. *Exp Eye Res*, **28**, 277–284
Saude, T. (1993) *Ocular Anatomy and Physiology*, Blackwell Scientific, Oxford, p. 140
Spooner, J.D. (1957) *Ocular Anatomy*, Hatton Press, London, pp. 115–117

43 Figure 3.5 shows a transverse section of the eye region of an embryo with three aspects marked I, II and III as well as seven features which are given letters A to G. Identify the most correct answers to each of the following.

(i)   Which aspect is the one most likely to be the surface: I, II or III?

(ii)   What is the most likely crown to rump length of the embryo: 2, 10, 20, 50, 90, 200, 400 or 4000 mm?

(iii)   What is the most likely age of the embryo: 1, 5, 20, 50, 90 or 200 weeks?

(iv)   Which letter (A to G) identifies the surface of the future cornea?

(v)   Which letter (A to G) identifies the future lens?

(vi)   Which letter (A to G) identifies the future vitreous?

(vii)   Which letter (A to G) identifies the sinus of Von Szily?

(viii) Which letter (A to G) identifies the neural part of the future retina?

(ix)   Which letter (A to G) is most likely to indicate the unclosed choroidal fissure?

(x)   Which letter (A to G) identifies the surface ectoderm?

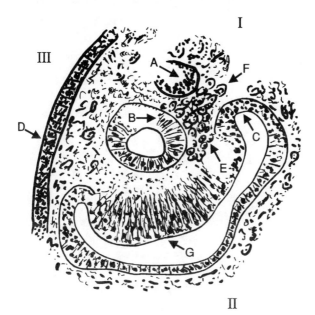

Fig. 3.5 Details of structures of an embryonic eye in transverse section.

43 (i) III; (ii) 10 mm; (iii) 5 weeks; (iv) D; (v) B; (vi) E; (vii) C; (viii) G; (ix) F; (x) D. *Note*: D is correct for two items but A is correct for none of these items.

References

Duke-Elder, W.S. (1932) *Textbook of Ophthalmology*, Kimpton, London, pp. 338–344

Snell, R.S. and Lemp, M.A. (1989) *Clinical Anatomy of the Eye*, Blackwell Scientific, Boston, pp. 1–7

Spooner, J.D. (1957) *Ocular Anatomy*, Hatton Press, London, pp. 148–159

Wolff, E. (1933) *The Anatomy of the Eye and Orbit*, Lewis, London, pp. 227–242

4 Contact lenses

1 An eye is satisfactorily corrected for hyperopia with a hard contact lens with a back vertex power in air of +1.50 DS, which has a back central optic radius of 7.70 mm. The lens is modified, increasing the back central optic radius to 7.75 mm. Which of the following is most likely to be required?

A The lens must also have the front surface changed to make the back vertex power in air more plus, after modification of the back surface to a flatter curve

B No power modification is needed, since the liquid lens will mask any possible difficulties over power

C A steeper front surface must be made, assuming that an insignificant change in thickness will be involved

D The front surface must be made flatter, to reduce its positive power, making the back vertex power of the modified lens in air less plus and compensating for the change of the back surface

2 In fitting contact lenses to a small infant, corneal radius and corneal diameter are of particular interest. Which of the following items is the one most likely to be true?

A Assuming an adult corneal radius to be 7.8 mm, the radius in late secondary infancy (approximately 5 years) is more likely to be 5.50 mm than 7.50 mm

B The refractive error of an aphakic infant may change from over +25 D in the early months of life to about +14 D some 4 years later

C The corneal diameter of an infant hardly alters over the first 4 years of life

D Direct profile photography of the cornea is more accurate than photokeratoscopy when measuring the corneal radius of an infant

4   Contact lenses: Answers

1   As shown in the example given in Fletcher *et al.* (1994), it is D which is most likely, since the (–) change in the front of the liquid lens is less than the (+) change in power of the back surface of the lens.

References

Douthwaite, W.A. (1987) *Contact Lens Optics*, Butterworths, London, pp. 36–46
Fletcher, R., Lupelli, L. and Rossi, A. (1994) *Contact Lens Practice*, Blackwell Scientific, Oxford, p. 233
Phillips, A.J. and Stone, J. (1989) *Contact Lenses*, 3rd edn, Butterworths, London, p. 219

2   Item D has been described by Kon (1991) as being of low accuracy. Item B is most likely; see Lupelli (1994). He also indicates that the value in A is more likely to be 7.50 mm than 5.50 mm. See also Speedwell (1989), who describes almost 2 mm increase in corneal diameter during the first year of life.

References

Kon, Y.P. (1991) Some methods of corneal measurement *Contact Lens J*, 19 (Suppl.), p. 2
Lupelli, L. (1994) In *Contact Lens Practice* (eds R. Fletcher, L. Lupelli and A. Rossi), Blackwell Scientific, Oxford, p. 239
Moore, B.D. (1989) Changes in the aphakic refraction of children with unilateral congenital cataracts. *J Pediatr Ophthalmol and Strabismus*, **26**, 290–295
Speedwell, L. (1989) In *Contact Lenses* (eds A.J. Phillips and J. Stone), Butterworths, London, p. 783

3 Keratoconus has long been an indication for the use of contact
lenses, and recently there has been increased interest in corneal
topography related to such conditions. Which one of the
following items do you consider to be most accurate?

A Vertical planes of light can be projected on to the cornea,
followed by computer analysis of the data obtained to
produce contour maps of nearly spherical corneas. The
technique is not suitable for irregular corneas such as are
found in keratoconus

B In keratoconus the cones tend to develop inferonasally, yet
they are sometimes found centrally or above centre

C High astigmatism is a very late feature of keratoconus

D Pellucid marginal corneal degeneration, which involves both
thinning and distortion of the cornea, is always found in the
superior part of the cornea

4 In hard contact lens fitting the liquid lens is an important optical
feature and some 'clinical rules' are often used (with some care)
when considering liquid lens changes. Assume that a hard corneal
lens afocal in air (for a distant object) has a back optic zone
radius (BOZR) of 8.00 mm and this lens exactly corrects an eye
which has a corneal radius of 7.90 mm. A second lens, also afocal
in air, is substituted but this one has a BOZR of 7.95 mm. Which
of the following is correct?

A The eye will be undercorrected for myopia by approximately
0.25 D

B A spectacle lens approximately +0.62 D will now be required,
in addition to the contact lens

C The eye will be fogged approximately 0.50 D

Contact lenses: Answers

3 Item B should be chosen as being most accurate; see Klyce (1993). Item D is incorrect as the thinning is of the inferior region; see Ostler and Ostler (1992). The ways in which items A and C are presented are virtually the opposite of what is described by de Cunha and Woodward (1993).

References
de Cunha, D. and Woodward, E.G. (1993) Measurement of corneal topography in keratoconus. *Ophthal Physiol Opt*, **13**, 377–382

Klyce, S.D. (1993) In *Excimer Laser Surgery* (eds F.B. Thompson and P.J. McDonnell), Igaku-Shion, New York, p. 33

Ostler, H.B. and Ostler, M.W. (1992) *Diseases of the External Eye and Adnexa*, Williams & Wilkins, Baltimore, pp. 233–234

4 Item A is correct. Assume a refractive index of 1.336 for the liquid, ignoring the contact lenses apart from their back surfaces which form the front of each liquid lens, you should assume that the cornea is always the same radius. Then the first liquid lens has a (fully corrective) power of $-0.53\,D$ (using $336/7.90 = -42.53\,D$ and $336/8.00 = +42.00\,D$) while the second liquid lens has a power of $-0.27\,D$.

References
Bennett, A.G. (1963) *Optics of Contact Lenses*, Assn. Disp. Opticians, London, pp. 25–29

Douthwaite, W.A. (1987) *Contact Lens Optics*, Butterworths, London, pp. 35–39 (in which note use of 'BCOR')

Fowler, C. (1994) In *Contact Lens Practice* (eds M. Ruben and M. Guillon), Chapman & Hall, London, p. 126

5 Movement of contact lenses is normally a feature influenced by
   fit and other factors. Which of the following items is most likely
   to be correct?

   A   During the first minute after insertion of a hydrogel lens one
       can predict with great certainty that the lens will be moving
       the same amount during blinking after 8 hours' wear
   B   Blinking with the eye in the primary position, some
       20 minutes after insertion of a soft lens, should produce about
       0.75 to 1 mm of vertical movement in a typical good fit
   C   Blinking with the eye looking well above the primary
       position is likely to reduce greatly the amount of vertical
       movement of a hydrogel lens
   D   The film of tears beneath a hard contact lens may influence
       the manner in which blinking causes the lens to move on the
       eye, but this tears film has no effect on the movement of a
       hydrogel lens on the eye

Contact lenses: Answers

5 Items A and D do not accurately reflect the conclusions of recent Australian observations. Item B is a reasonable choice, while C tends to contradict commonly accepted observations.

References
Brennan, N.A. *et al.* (1994) Soft lens movement: temporal characteristics. *Optometry and Vision Science*, **71**, 359–363

Guillon, M. (1994) In *Contact Lens Practice* (eds M. Ruben and M. Guillon), Chapman & Hall, London, pp. 561 and 598–599

Little, S.L. and Bruce, A.S. (1994) Hydrogel (Acuvue) lens movement is influenced by postlens tear film. *Optometry and Vision Science*, **71**, 364–370

Rossi, A. (1994) In *Contact Lens Practice* (Fletcher, R., Lupelli, L. and Rossi, A.), Blackwell Scientific, Oxford, p. 150

6 The method described first by Drysdale in 1900 is commonly used to measure the radius of the back surface of a contact lens. Figure 4.1 shows the original method using a distant object, but a target such as that shown as T can be used near the beam-splitter BS. Which of the following suggestions is most likely to be correct?

A Assuming a relaxed emmetropic observer, the microscope should not be in infinity focus

B The distance D through which the lens surface is moved for radius measurement is twice the actual radius, since light reaches position A and is reflected

C Any scratches on the surface should be noticed in focus at the same time, as position B also brings the target into focus

D Hydrogel lenses (when hydrated) cannot be measured by this technique, since they would have to be suspended in saline

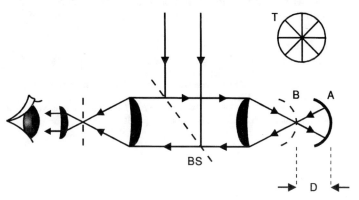

Fig. 4.1 The principle of a well-known system for measurement of contact lens surfaces.

7 A disinfection or 'D' value is sometimes noted as a time for reducing organisms in a solution to a certain level. Which of the following statements is most appropriate or accurate?

A D values can be applied directly to the effects of cleaning contact lenses by rubbing and rinsing

B D values are useful for quantitative comparisons of solutions used for disinfection

C D values do not assume constancy of the time for reducing contamination throughout the whole disinfection process

D Clinical performance of a solution can be based on D values, ignoring factors relating to bacterial or fungal contamination

Contact lenses: Answers

6 Items A and B should be dismissed on basic optical considerations. Item C is in accord with common practice and should be chosen. Item D, happily, is not correct provided that the submerged lens is supported suitably and a very strong light is used; however, steps must be taken to mask reflections from the surface which are not of interest.

References

Bier, N. and Lowther, G.E. (1977) *Contact Lens Correction*, Butterworths, London, pp. 232–235

Drysdale, C.V. (1900) On a simple method of determining the curvatures of small lenses. *Trans Opt Soc*, 1–12

Fletcher, R., Lupelli, L. and Rossi, A. (1994) *Contact Lens Practice*, Blackwell Scientific, Oxford, pp. 110–111 and 124–125

Ruben, M. and Guillon, M. (1994) *Contact Lens Practice*, Chapman & Hall, London, pp. 150–154 and 174

7 Item B should be chosen; although the D value does indicate performance under a laboratory regime, it allows comparisons.

References

Fleiszig, M.J. *et al.* (1992) In *Clinical Contact Lens Practice* (eds E.S. Bennett and B.A. Weissman), Lippincott, Philadelphia, Ch. 36, p. 17

Lowe, R. *et al.* (1992) Comparative efficacy of contact lens disinfection solutions. *CLAO Journal*, **18**, 34–40

Stapleton, F. and Stechler, J. (1994) In *Contact Lens Practice* (eds M. Ruben and M. Guillon), Chapman & Hall, London, p. 536

8 The term Dk/t is now familiar as an important feature of the design and selection of contact lenses. Which of the following is most correctly associated with the term?

A Wetting, usually as indicated by *contact angle*
B A dioptric change in the cornea, related to the speed of change
C Diffusion of liquid through the cornea, divided by time
D Oxygen transmissibility of a contact lens at its centre

9 Fluorescein is commonly used for photography in optometric practice. Which of the following combinations of filters is best for this photography?

A A filter over the illuminant which does not pass radiation between 350 and 500 nm, with a blue barrier filter over the camera lens
B A blue filter (perhaps Wratten 47, 47A or 47B) over the illuminant and a light yellow filter over the camera lens
C An ultraviolet absorbing filter over the illuminant and a medium red filter over the camera
D A filter passing chiefly light of wavelength about 640 nm over the illuminant and one passing chiefly about 330 nm over the camera lens

10 A chronic oedematous corneal condition known as bullous keratopathy can often be alleviated by a contact lens. Which of the following suggestions is likely to be most suitable?

A The epithelial bullae may be minimized by contact lenses but there is seldom any lessening of pain and blepharospasm
B The persistent pain associated with the condition is best controlled by a hard contact lens fitted small and steep
C A bandage lens with a high water content (perhaps tinted) can be provided for extended wear even though this could possibly be lost during sleep
D A low water content hydrogel lens is most suitable but if the oedema is confined to the corneal epithelium, visual acuity is unlikely to be improved

8 Item B should be recognized as perhaps the most absurd of three untruths! It is correct to select D, as will be supported by the following references, bearing in mind that the form 'Dk/L' has been used and now tends to be superceded.

References

Benjamin, W.J. (1994) In *Contact Lens Practice* (eds M. Ruben and M. Guillon), Chapman & Hall, London, p. 48

Loran, D.F.C. (1989) In *Contact Lenses* (eds A.J. Phillips and J. Stone), Butterworths, London, pp. 487–488

Lupelli, L. (1994) In *Contact Lens Practice* (R. Fletcher, L. Lupelli and A. Rossi), Blackwell Scientific, Oxford, p. 24

9 Item B represents a typical recommendation and the other suggestions are all inappropriate.

References

Bishop, C. (1976) Basic aspects of ophthalmic photography. *Optician*, **16**, 719

Henson, D.B. (1983) *Optometric Instrumentation*, Butterworths, London, p. 142

Long, W.F. (1991) In *Clinical Procedures in Optometry* (eds J.B. Eskridge *et al.*), Lippincott, Philadelphia, pp. 326 and 634

Lupelli, L. (1994) In *Contact Lens Practice* (R. Fletcher, L. Lupelli and A. Rossi), Blackwell Scientific, Oxford, pp. 74–75

10 The item of choice is C, as should be supported by the references below.

References

Astin, C.L.K. (1991) Therapeutic contact lenses – an overview of some lens types. *JBCLA*, **14**, 129–133

Gasset, A. and Kaufman, H. (1970) Bandage lenses in the treatment of bullous keratopathy. *Am J Ophthalmol*, **72**, 376–380

Rehim, M.H.A. and Samy, M. (1989) The role of therapeutic soft contact lenses in treatment of bullous keratopathy. *Contact Lens J*, **17**, 119–125

11 Figure 4.2 shows part of a hard contact lens with its axis of symmetry. It has a back central optic zone of one radius, which has a centre of curvature C2 and after a transition there is a peripheral zone with a longer radius. Which of the following terms correctly refers to the dimension here shown as ×?

A   Axial edge lift
B   Radial edge thickness
C   Carrier junction thickness
D   Radial edge lift

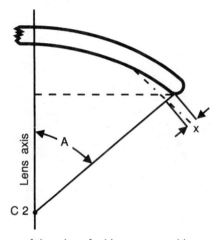

Fig. 4.2 Features of the edge of a bicurve corneal lens.

Contact lenses: Answers

11 The correct term is *radial edge lift*, as in BS 3521: Part 3: (1988). The line shown from C2, at an angle A to the lens axis, is the radius along which the radial edge lift is measured.

References

Fletcher, R., Lupelli, L. and Rossi, A. (1994) *Contact Lens Practice*, Blackwell Scientific, Oxford, pp. 39–40

Phillips, A.J. and Stone, J. (eds) (1989) *Contact Lenses*, Butterworths, London, p. 453

12 Soft contact lens wearing regimes have been the subject of several studies which have revealed distinct trends relating to the success and possible disadvantages of various approaches. Which of the following suggestions is most likely to be accurate?

A   The relative risk of developing keratitis is decreased if soft lenses are worn overnight

B   Wearers of disposable soft lenses, the use of which is restricted to daytime only, have more prevalent complications such as conjunctivitis than wearers of conventional daily wear soft lenses

C   Ocular dryness symptoms tend to be greater with disposable daily wear soft lenses than with non-disposable daily wear soft lenses. However, a sensation of grittiness is less common with the disposable lenses

D   The extent to which a patient is compliant to the instructions given by a practitioner, including frequent after-care examination, bears no relationship to the incidence of corneal infection associated with the wearing of soft contact lenses

13 Presbyopic corrections with contact lenses have been provided by an optical feature which tends to loss of contrast in the retinal image. However, the feature is likely to provide good vision for close objects which are above and below the primary position of the eye. Which of the following is most likely to describe a contact lens approach which uses the feature?

A   Diffractive bifocals in both eyes

B   Crescent bifocal with truncation in both eyes

C   Fused, straight-top segments in both eyes

D   Alternating vision, using undercorrection for near vision in one eye

Contact lenses: Answers

12 Item C has the support of at least one recent study. The other items do not reflect accurately accumulated experience.

References

Dart, J.K.G., Stapleton, F. and Minassian, D. (1991) Contact lenses and other risk factors in microbial keratitis. *Lancet*, **338**, 650–653

Fletcher, R., Lupelli, L. and Rossi, A. (1994) *Contact Lens Practice*, Blackwell Scientific, Oxford, p. 185

Kenyon, K.R. and John, T. (1994) In *Contact Lens Practice* (eds M. Ruben and M. Guillon), Chapman & Hall, London, pp. 1076–1081

Poggio, E.C. and Abelson, M.B. (1993) Complications and symptoms with disposable daily wear contact lenses and conventional soft daily wear contact lenses. *CLAOJ*, **19**, 95–102

13 Item A is most likely, although D might be a possibility in certain instances. Also the performance characteristics described could possibly be found with the use of certain of the aspheric surface designs, in which cases the contrast loss factor might be expected to be rather less evident.

References

Ruben, M. and Guillon, M. (1994) *Contact Lens Practice*, Chapman & Hall, London, pp. 135 and 778–779

Saunders, B.D. (1990) A soft diffractive bifocal contact lens. *Optician*, **200**, 15–18

14 A certain contact lens material has been described as being flexible, durable and resilient. It has a high permeability to oxygen. Fluorescein can be used when assessing the fit of contact lenses made from this material. During use it can incline corneal lenses to become 'tight'. It is basically hydrophobic and usually requires surface treatment to overcome this. Which of the following best describes this material?

A Hydroxyethylmethacrylate (HEMA)
B Styrene
C Filcon
D Silicone elastomer

15 The extent and the functions of the precorneal tears liquid must be considered in relation to certain symptoms; these symptoms may or may not be associated with the wearing of contact lenses. Which *two* of the following suggestions are most likely to be correct?

A Peripheral corneal desiccation is usually found at the top of the cornea (12 o'clock) as the result of wearing a hard corneal lens
B The height of the normal meniscus of tears liquid, viewed under the microscope, is likely to be between 0.1 and 0.4 mm
C Lack of tears, resulting in a slightly (marginally) dry eye is most often found in young adults with relatively long tears break up times
D Oedema of the corneal epithelium may result from prolonged swimming in a freshwater lake, with or without the use of contact lenses

Contact lenses: Answers

14 Item D is correct.

References

Fletcher, R., Lupelli, L. and Rossi, A. (1994) *Contact Lens Practice*, Blackwell
  Scientific, Oxford, pp. 17–21
Lowther, G.E. (1991) Contact lens performance considerations.
  In *Considerations in Contact Lens Use Under Adverse Conditions*
  (ed. P.E. Flatteau), National Academy Press, Washington, DC,
  pp. 131–132
Phillips, A.J. and Stone, J. (1989) *Contact Lenses*, 3rd edn, Butterworths,
  London, p. 363

15 Items B and D should be chosen.

References

Caffery, B.E. (1992) The dry eye? *J Br C L Ass*, **15**, 145–148
Fletcher, R., Lupelli, L. and Rossi, A. (1994) *Contact Lens Practice*, Blackwell
  Scientific, Oxford, pp. 98, 106 and 115
Port, M.J.A. and Asaria, T.S. (1990) The assessment of human tear volume.
  J Br C L Ass, **13**, 76–82

6 Hard (polymethylmethacrylate [PMMA] or gas permeable) contact lenses are capable of flexure under some circumstances (although the term rigid is sometimes used). This flexure may be on the eye or perhaps when badly stored in a restrictive case. Which of the following statements is most likely to be correct?

A The flexibility of a hard corneal lens with a central thickness of 0.14 mm is likely to increase by about 7% if the thickness is reduced to 0.07 mm

B Gas permeable corneal lenses tend to flex much less than PMMA lenses with very similar dimensions, such as thickness and total diameter as well as power

C A thin, flexible lens which tends to take up the shape of a very toroidal cornea during use will usually enhance visual acuity on account of the induced power changes

D Corneal lenses which have an elliptical back surface tend to flex less than those with an aspherical back surface

7 Hard corneal lenses intended for fitting, diagnostic assessment or issue from inventory stock may be stored either dry or in a soaking solution. Which of the following items is least likely to be correct?

A Wet storage permits disinfection of the lens
B Wet storage causes unfavourable instability of lens dimensions
C Wet storage favours surface wetting when the lens is removed and used
D It is possible that a container may be thought to be empty, unless carefully inspected

8 Contact lenses of different materials, forms, powers and thicknesses differ in dimensional stability. Which of the following is most likely?

A Lenses made of CAB flatten less than fluorosiloxane–acrylate lenses

B A dry PMMA corneal lens with a back vertex power of +15.00 DS, after overnight soaking, probably flattens twice as much as the flattening of a PMMA lens of −15.00 DS

C The back surface of a dry PMMA corneal lens with a back vertex power of −10.00 DS must be expected to flatten after overnight soaking

D A series of fissures, known as 'crazing' or 'cracking', is a back surface phenomenon found more often in PMMA lenses than in gas permeable hard lenses

16 Item D is most correct. Suggestions A and B are deliberately misleading. Item C is often questionable, particularly if the cornea has against-the-rule toricity.

References
Guillon, M. and Sammons, W.A. (1994) In *Contact Lens Practice* (eds M. Ruber and M. Guillon), Chapman & Hall, London, p. 100

Lupelli, L. (1994) In *Contact Lens Practice* (R. Fletcher, L. Lupelli and A. Rossi), Blackwell Scientific, Oxford, p. 100

Stevenson, R.W.W. (1988) Flexibility of hard gas permeable contact lenses. *Am J Optom Physiol Optics*, **65**, 874–879

17 Item B is probably *least* likely. Changes are likely to take place when the lens is soaked but these will settle and will produce the state most likely during wear. Drying of the solution should be avoided.

References
Fletcher, R., Lupelli, L. and Rossi, A. (1994) *Contact Lens Practice*, Blackwell Scientific, Oxford, pp. 31, 52 and 96

Gordon, S. (1965) Contact lens hydration: a study of the wetting cycle. *Optom Weekly*, **56**, 55–62

18 Item C is correct. There is some error in each of the other items, which may not be apparent at first!

References
Fletcher, R., Lupelli, L. and Rossi, A. (1994) *Contact Lens Practice*, Blackwell Scientific, Oxford, pp. 31 and 96

Pearson, R.M. (1978) Dimensional stability of lathe cut CAB lenses. *J Am Optom Ass*, **49**, 927–929

Phillips, A.J. (1969) Contact lens plastics, solutions and storage – some implications. *Ophthal Optician*, **9**, 75–79

Phillips, A.J. and Stone, J. (1989) *Contact Lenses*, 3rd edn, Butterworths, London, p. 135

19 Scleral lenses, very useful in some circumstances, have fitting and power features somewhat different from those peculiar to hard corneal lenses. Which of the following is most likely to be correct?

A   To achieve optimum features of the liquid lens and air bubble behind a fenestrated scleral lens, central corneal clearance is critical; this should be 0.4 to 0.5 mm after settling

B   While a preformed scleral lens should have a BOZR about 0.15 mm steeper than the steepest corneal meridian, the BOZR of a lens made from an eye impression must be about 2.25 mm flatter than this

C   If a BOZR of 8.50 mm at first appears to be what should be ordered for a new scleral lens, but some doubt exists, it is better to order a BOZR of 8.40 mm

D   A scleral lens should be cleaned before use but a wetting solution must never be used

20 Deposits which build up, or impacted foreign bodies on corneal lenses may cause certain problems for wearers and this is very significant for hydrogel lenses. Which of the following is most likely to be correct?

A   Any immunological response to materials bound to a soft lens cannot be attributed to protein deposits

B   Proteins in the tears are less likely to produce deposits on non-ionic contact lens materials with a low water content than on ionic (high water) materials

C   Thermal disinfection of HEMA lenses, which are seldom replaced, is the best method to use for disinfecting such lenses

D   Slit lamp examination of soft lenses is highly satisfactory for the early detection of protein deposits, although these never appear during the first month of wear

Contact lenses: Answers

19 Item C is correct.

References
Bier, N. (1957) *Contact Lens Practice*, 2nd edn, Butterworth Scientific, London, p. 48

Fletcher, R., Lupelli, L. and Rossi, A. (1994) *Contact Lens Practice*, Blackwell Scientific, Oxford, pp. 205–207 and 211–212

Pullum, K.W. (1989) In *Contact Lenses* (eds A.J. Phillips and J. Stone), Butterworths, London, p. 665

20 Item B is the best choice, some of the others being questionable or even incorrect.

References
Fletcher, R., Lupelli, L. and Rossi, A. (1994) *Contact Lens Practice*, Blackwell Scientific, Oxford, p. 164

Grant, T. *et al.* (1989) Contact lens related papillary conjunctivitis (CLPC): influence of protein accumulation and replacement frequency. *Invest Ophthalmol Vis Sci*, **30** (Suppl.), p. 166

Lin, S.T. *et al.* (1991) Protein accumulation on disposable extended wear lenses. *CLAOJ*, **17**, 44–50

Sack, Z , Jones, B. and Antignani, A. (1987) Specificity and biological activity of the protein deposited on the hydrogel surface. *Invest Ophthalmol Vis Sci*, **28**, 842–849

21 Hydrogen peroxide is a well established disinfectant for hydrogel contact lenses. Which *two* of the following suggestions are correct and which are incorrect?

A   A patient has no symptoms using a soft lens previously disinfected with hydrogen peroxide. There cannot be any possible danger to the corneal epithelium

B   A platinum disc, used as an adjunct to neutralization of hydrogen peroxide after disinfecting a soft lens, acts extremely rapidly

C   The safe use of hydrogen peroxide in disinfecting soft lenses involves considerable neutralization of this disinfectant

D   Fairly high amounts of hydrogen peroxide, capable of potential damage, can be left in contact lenses after some 'neutralization' procedures

22 Without a contact lens correction most eyes demonstrate some spherical aberration, which may affect visual performance. Several studies have addressed the question as to whether contact lenses influence ocular spherical aberration and its effects. Which of the following suggestions is most likely to be correct?

A   Contact lenses can significantly alter the ocular spherical aberration and, even when that is less than 1 D, the change drastically reduces visual acuity

B   The crystalline lens significantly reduces the spherical aberration of the unaccommodated eye and when accommodating tends to increase spherical aberration

C   Ocular spherical aberration can be measured during the use of either hard or soft contact lenses, showing that there is little difference in each situation

23 Which of the following characteristics is/are *not* true of hydrogen peroxide, when compared to other cold disinfection systems?

A   There is a reduced risk of an allergic response

B   There is an increased risk of an allergic response

C   It requires no preservative

D   It may be used without rinsing prior to insertion of the lenses

21 The last two items, C and D may be regarded as correct, certainly with a view to being cautious.

References

Fletcher, R., Lupelli, L. and Rossi, A. (1994) *Contact Lens Practice*, Blackwell Scientific, Oxford, p. 165

Gyulai, P. *et al.* (1987) Relative neutralization ability of six hydrogen peroxide disinfection systems. *Contact Lens Spectrum*, **2**, 61–68

Tripathi, B.J. and Tripathi, R.C. (1989) Hydrogen peroxide damage to human corneal epithelial cells *in vitro*. *Arch Ophthalmol*, **107**, 1516–1519

22 Item C is the correct one, the others being misleading.

References

Collins, M.J., Brown, B. and Atchison, D.A. (1992) Tolerance to spherical aberration induced by rigid contact lenses. *Ophthal Physiol Opt*, **12**, 24–28

Millodot, M. and Sivak, J.G. (1974) Measurement of the spherical aberration of the crystalline lens *in vivo*, a preliminary report. *Atti Fond G Ronchi*, **29**, 903–908

Woo, G.C.S. and Sivak, J.G. (1976) The effect of hard and soft contact lenses (Soflens™) on the spherical aberration of the human eye. *Am J Optom Physiol Opt*, **53**, 459–463

23 B and D are correct. Hydrogen peroxide (H_2O_2) breaks down to H_2O and O_2 when exposed to a catalyst (e.g. a platinum disc), thus reducing the likelihood of causing allergic reaction. Alternatively, exposure to sodium pyruvate results in the production of sodium acetate, water and CO_2 which is in turn dissolved in the solution. This allows for simpler case design as there is no resulting build-up of pressure.

   The catalysts chosen to break down the H_2O_2 are generally present in the tears and thus unlikely to cause an allergic response although in some formulations, preservatives may be required, again risking such a response.

Reference

Phillips, A.J. and Stone, J. (1989) *Contact Lenses*, 3rd edn, Butterworths, London, pp. 144–146

24 Which of the following is most true of the normal corneal contour?

   A   Flattens from centre to periphery
   B   Steepens from centre to periphery
   C   Flattens from centre to periphery, rate of flattening being greatest nasally
   D   Flattens from centre to periphery, rate of flattening being greatest temporally
   E   Steepens from centre to periphery, rate of steepening being greatest temporally

25 There have been various conventions concerning the naming of the specifications of contact lenses. Which of the following acronyms do/does not refer to the back optic zone radius?

   A   BC
   B   BCOR
   C   PCCR
   D   BCOD

26 A patient with a spectacle correction of –20 DS, BVD 10 mm is to be fitted with contact lenses. What will the ocular refraction be (rounded to the nearest dioptre)?

   A   –10 DS
   B   –17 DS
   C   –20 DS
   D   –25 DS
   E   –30 DS

27 A 20 dioptre hyperope is to be fitted with contact lenses, BVD 10 mm. What will the ocular refraction be (rounded to the nearest dioptre)?

   A   +10 DS
   B   +17 DS
   C   +20 DS
   D   +25 DS
   E   +30 DS

Contact lenses: Answers

24 C is most true: the normal cornea flattens from centre to periphery, rate of flattening being greatest nasally.

References

Bier, N. (1959) *Contact Lens Routine and Practice*, 2nd edn, pp. 127–130
Holladay, J.T. and Waring, G.O.(III) (1992) Optics and topography of radial keratotomy. In *Refractive Keratotomy* (ed. G.O. Waring (III)), Mosby, St Louis, pp. 91–97
Maguire, L.J. (1988) Corneal topography. In *The Cornea* (eds H.E. Kaufman *et al.*), Churchill Livingstone, New York, pp. 897–908

25 D is correct. BCOD stands for back central optic diameter, and refers to the size of the central zone, not its radius of curvature. BC stands for base curve (use is limited to spectacle lenses in the UK; occasionally used elsewhere for contact lenses), BCOR for back central optic radius and PCCR for central posterior curve radius (this is not used in British contact lens practice).

Reference

Lowther, G.E. and Snyder, C. (1992) *Contact Lenses Procedures and Techniques*, 2nd edn, Butterworths, Boston, p. 17

26 B is correct.

References

Bennett, A.G. (1985) *Optics of Contact Lens*, 3rd edn, Association of Dispensing Opticians, pp. 7 and 89
Douthwaite, W.A. (1987) *Contact Lens Optics*, Butterworths, London, pp. 1–3

27 D is correct.

References

Bennett, A.G. (1985) *Optics of Contact Lens*, 3rd edn, Association of Dispensing Opticians, pp. 7 and 89
Douthwaite, W.A. (1987) *Contact Lens Optics*, Butterworths, London, pp. 1–3

28 Which of the following statements is *incorrect* concerning the oxygen requirements of the cornea?

A 8% oxygen is available to the cornea during eye closure
B The normal partial pressure of oxygen at sea level is 159 mmHg
C Corneal swelling occurs only when the available oxygen drops to below 4% at sea level
D Corneal sensitivity is reduced if the precorneal oxygen tension drops to below 8%

29 Which of the following statements is *incorrect* concerning the microbe acanthamoeba?

A Acanthamoeba can exist in two forms – the cyst and the trophozoite
B Acanthamoeba can survive at temperatures ranging from –22°C to 42°C
C Acanthaemoeba is a rare organism found only in stagnant water
D Acanthamoeba can survive in solutions whose pHs range from 3.9 to 9.75

30 Which of the following disinfectants is most reliable in the elimination of acanthamoeba?

A Chlorine
B Hydrogen peroxide
C Chlorhexidine
D Heat

Contact lenses: Answers

28 C is incorrect as corneal swelling can occur at oxygen levels higher than this. Generally it is felt that 10% oxygen (i.e. a partial pressure of 76 mmHg) is required to avoid corneal swelling. Approximately 21% of the air is oxygen, thus at normal sea level pressure of 1 atmosphere = 760 mmHg; 21% of this pressure is 160 mmHg.

Reference

Tomlinson, A. (1992) Oxygen requirements of the cornea. In *Complications of Contact Lens Wear* (ed. A. Tomlinson), Mosby-Year Book, St Louis, pp. 6–8

29 C is incorrect. Acanthamoeba is in fact extremely common, being found in air and all kinds of water including chlorinated swimming pools.

References

Ashton, N. and Stamm, W. (1975) Amoebic infection of the eye. A pathological report. *Trans Ophthalmol Soc UK*, **95**, 214–220
Buckley, R.J. (1991) Acanthamoeba in perspective. *J BCLA*, **14**, 5–7
Cohen, E.J. *et al.* (1985) Diagnosis and management of acanthamoeba keratitis. *Am J Ophthalmol*, **100**, 389–395
Moore, M.B. (1990) Acanthamoeba keratitis and contact lens wear: the patient is at fault. *Cornea*, **9** (Suppl. 1), S33–S35

30 D is correct. Heat is most reliable as long as temperatures of >65°C have been maintained for more than 5½ minutes and 70°C for at least 1 minute.

References

Larkin, D.F.P. (1991) In *Contact Lenses* (eds G. Smolin and M.H. Friedlander), *International Ophthalmology Clinics*, **31**(2), pp. 163–172
Phillips, A.J. and Stone, J. (1989) *Contact Lenses*, 3rd edn, Butterworths, London, p. 142

5 Drug uses and actions for optometrists

1 The following items concern the topical use of a local anaesthetic solution, for example in optometric practice. Which one is correct?

    A   Benoxinate usually produces corneal anaesthesia adequate for applanation tonometry within 60 sec

    B   Diffuse epithelial desquamation, which may reduce visual acuity to 6/20, may follow the application of benoxinate

    C   A local anaesthetic solution such as benoxinate, applied to the cornea, has no effect on corneal permeability

    D   Most topical local anaesthetics tend to retard healing of any defects of the corneal epithelium

    E   Benoxinate, in concentrations even lower than 0.4%, may produce adequate very short-term decrease of corneal sensitivity for some purposes

2 Despite some reported side effects, cyclopentolate remains in some favour as a mydriatic and cycloplegic. Choose the one item below which is actually the most correct statement.

    A   Cyclopentolate hydrochloride (1%) is unsuitable for administration, for example to children, by spray onto eyelids which are temporarily closed

    B   Cyclopentolate hydrochloride (1%) is not likely to produce mydriasis or cycloplegia within 1 hour but full recovery is as rapid as the effect

    C   Cyclopentolate hydrochloride (0.5%) is likely to produce mydriasis more slowly than 0.5% tropicamide, and recovery time (for cyclopentolate) would probably be longer

    D   Cyclopentolate hydrochloride is essentially an adrenergic agent

5 Drug uses and actions for optometrists: Answers

1 Item C is incorrect and should be chosen, since there is an acute disruption of epithelial paracellular junctions, altering permeability; see Klyce and Beurman (1988). Smith (1984) indicated the correctness of A. Bartlett and Jaanus (1989) support the reliability of B and of E and Johnson and Forest (1994) agree with D.

References
Bartlett, J.D. and Jaanus, S.D. (1989) *Clinical Ocular Pharmacology*, 2nd edn, Butterworths, Boston, pp. 154–156
Johnson, R.W. and Forrest, F.C. (1994) *Local and General Anaesthesia for Ophthalmic Surgery*, Butterworth-Heinemann, Oxford, p. 42
Klyce, S.D. and Beurman, R.W. (1988) In *The Cornea* (eds H.E. Kaufman *et al.*), Churchill Livingstone, New York
Smith, M.B. (1984) *Handbook of Ocular Pharmacology*, 3rd edn

2 The only correct item is C, which can be substantiated by reference to Bartlett and Jaanus (1989, p. 129) and Miller (1987, p. 50). See the same references concerning item B; also Miller (1987, p. 50) and Bartlett and Jaanus (1989, p. 132) for item D.

Vale and Cox (1985) should also be noted. Item A can be followed up in Ismail (1994) where the spray method was found to be easy and effective.

References
Bartlett, J.D. and Jaanus, S.D. (1989) *Clinical Ocular Pathology*, Butterworths, Boston
Ismail, E.E. *et al.* (1994) A comparison of drop installation and spray application of 1% cyclopentolate hydrochloride. *Optometry and Vision Science*, **71**, 235–241
Miller, S. (1987) *Clinical Ophthalmology*, Wright, London
Vale, J. and Cox, B. (1985) *Drugs and the Eye*, 2nd edn, Butterworths, London, pp. 31–32 and 34

3 A child aged 4 years has no apparent binocular problems and has unaided vision of 6/5 in each eye but is given a refractive examination after 0.5% atropine has been administered correctly over the previous 3 days. Which of the following suggestions is most satisfactory, assuming that the cycloplegic refraction is R + 1.50 DS/−0.25 DC × 20; L +1.25 DS and that no symptoms have been reported?

   A   Allowing 0.50 D on account of ciliary tonus, add this +0.50 D to the cycloplegic data and prescribe for constant wear R +2.00/−0.25 × 20; L +1.75 DS

   B   Making a deduction of +1.00 DS for tonus and ignoring the small residual error, discharge without any prescription for spectacles, suggesting a routine check-up in 18 months

   C   Inform the parents that no spectacles are needed, apart from use of sunspectacles for 1 extra day only, and that the pupils can be expected to return to normal next morning and reading should again be easy the next evening

   D   Suggest that the child should be re-examined, again under atropine, in 1 month

4 One per cent cyclopentolate has been administered as a cycloplegic to a 10-year-old girl who appears to teachers and parents to be myopic. Which of the following items do you judge to be the most appropriate?

   A   Since the refractive correction, after allowances for tonus, appears to be R and L +0.50/−1.25 × 180, giving good visual acuity, this is what is prescribed, requesting return in 6 months

   B   The raw refractive correction, without tonus allowance, is R +0.50/−1.25 × 180 = 6/6; L +0.25/−1.00 × 180 = 6/6 and no spectacles should be prescribed

   C   Hoping to prevent progression of suspected myopia, the correction suggested under A is given, but in bifocal form with a +2.75 DS addition each eye, with high segments, for constant use

   D   The cycloplegic is given at 14.15 hours, soon after arrival, and the refractive examination is commenced immediately so that it is completed, apart from ophthalmoscopy, by 14.25 hours

3 At this age, with the absence of difficulties described, item B should be a reasonable choice.

References
Bartlett, J.D. and Jaanus, S.D. (1989) *Clinical Ocular Pharmacology*, Butterworths, Boston, pp. 426–428

Mitchell, D.W.A. (1960) In *The Principles and Practice of Refraction* (ed. G.H. Giles), Hammond and Hammond, London, pp. 581–585

Press, L.J. and Moore, B.D. (1993) *Clinical Pediatric Optometry*, Butterworth-Heinemann, Boston, p. 352

Zetterstrom, C. (1985) A cross over study of the cycloplegic effects of a single topical application of cyclopentolate-phenylephrine and routine atropinization for 3.5 days. *Acta Ophthal*, **63**, 525–529

4 Item A is the most satisfactory, according to most informed opinions.

References
Scheiman, M.M. and Rouse, M.W. (1994) *Optometric Management of Learning-Related Disorders*, Mosby, St Louis, p. 269

Shakespeare, A.R. (1993) In *Visual Problems in Childhood* (ed. T. Buckingham), Butterworth-Heinemann, Oxford, pp. 233–236

5 It is sometimes appropriate to dilate a patient's pupils. In this connection, which of the following suggestions is most correct?

   A It is unwise to use a mydriatic on anyone over the age of 40 years
   B It is a legal requirement that all patients shall be informed in writing of possible hazards from 'angle closure' before mydriasis is attempted
   C The use of a miotic after mydriasis is completely without risk
   D The risk of angle closure from a mydriatic is small since it has been estimated that such closure in a normal population is likely in less than one person in about 18 000 or 20 000

6 Chloroquine has been used in the medical treatment of several conditions and has some recognized ocular unwanted effects. Which of the following short lists is the most appropriate in this connection?

   A Keratopathy, possibly with reversible opacities; retinopathy with colour vision defects
   B Miosis and ptosis
   C Black grains deposited in the palpebral conjunctiva and/or thick, advanced pinquecula
   D Deposits of gold salts in the lens, often following the sutures

7 Chloramphenicol is considered to be effective against many bacteria but while three of the following can be considered to be correct, you should identify the one which is not correct.

   A The drug has a toxic effect which is proportional to the dose given
   B The drug can pass both the blood–brain barrier and the blood–aqueous barrier
   C It is considered to be very effective against *Pseudomonas aeruginosa*
   D Extensive systemic therapy is seldom continued for more than a week

191

5 The first three items have significant difficulties. While C may be the subject of some differences of opinion, it is best considered to be incorrect, as stated. Thus D is the item which should be chosen.

References

Brown, F.G. and Fletcher, R. (1990) *Glaucoma in Optometric Practice*, Blackwell Scientific, Oxford, pp. 23–25

Classe, J.G. (1989) *Legal Aspects of Optometry*, Butterworths, Boston, pp. 308–309

Keller, J.T. (1975) The risk of angle closure from the use of mydriatics. *J Am Optom Ass*, **46**, 19–21

6 The last item refers rather to lenticular chrysiasis from gold salts which, like chloroquine, are sometimes also used in rheumatoid arthritis. Items B and C are misleading and incorrect suggestions. Item A should be chosen.

References

Bartlett, J.D. and Jaanus, S.D. (1989) *Clinical Ocular Pharmacology*, 2nd edn, Butterworths, Boston, pp. 803–804

Gittinger, J.W. and Asdourian, G.K. (1988) *Manual of Clinical Problems in Ophthalmology*, Little, Brown, Boston, pp. 140–141

Jaeger, W. and Krastel, H. (1987) Colour vision deficiencies caused by pharmacotherapy. In *Colour Vision Deficiencies*, VIII (ed. G. Verriest), Junk, Dordrecht, pp. 37–52

Nauman, G.O.H. and Apple, D.J. (1985) *Pathology of the Eye*, Springer, New York, pp. 388–389; 616; 627

7 The incorrect statement, which should be identified as such, is C.

References

Bartlett, J.D. and Jaanus, S.D. (1989) *Clinical Ocular Pharmacology*, Butterworths, Boston, pp. 221 and 853

British College of Optometrists (1994) *Optometrist's Formulary*, No. 2, London, p. 20

Ostler, H.B. (1992) *Diseases of the External Eye and Adnexa*, Williams & Wilkins, Baltimore, p. 802

Ruben, M. and Guillon, M. (1994) *Contact Lens Practice*, Chapman & Hall, London, p. 545

Taylor, S.P. and Austen, D.P. (1992) *Law and Management in Optometric Practice*, 2nd edn, Butterworth-Heinemann, Oxford, pp. 104–105

8 You are informed that a patient with slight anisochoria (right pupil smaller) was investigated at hospital as follows. After some seconds in relative darkness both pupils dilated, the left one normally and the right one less. Relatively strong sympathomimetic eye drops were instilled (right and left) and after 30 minutes the left pupil was dilated much more than the right pupil. Which of the following suggestions is most likely?

    A Probably Adie's pupil was present
    B The eye drops could have been cyclopentolate
    C A parasympathetic innervation disorder was present
    D The patient could have Horner's syndrome

9 A popular beta-blocker (beta-adrenergic antagonist) timolol is used as topical eye drops. Which one of the following items is the only correct one?

    A The amount of timolol in the plasma, 1 hour after 0.5% timolol has been dropped into the conjunctival sac, is less when punctal occlusion is present than when the puncta are free
    B Timolol administered as eye drops has several possible side effects, including a significant increase in heart rate in most people.
    C Timolol eye drops (used alone) dilate the pupil and therefore are not used in the control of raised intraocular pressure
    D Timolol eye drops tend to cause an increase in the production of aqueous humour at the site of the ciliary epithelium

10 Various drugs have been tried in the management of myopia, for example to attempt to reduce increases in myopia during youth or even in adulthood. Which *two* of the following statements are most likely to be correct?

    A Pilocarpine might slightly halt the progression of myopia by reducing intraocular pressure
    B Since accommodation may increase axial length (over a period of time), tropicamide has been given to some subjects at night, to reduce any ciliary spasm
    C Daily application of atropine has given no encouragement that this might delay progression of myopia
    D A mydriatic would improve the retinal image and increase the likelihood of a reduction in progression of myopia

Drug uses and actions for optometrists: Answers

8 The first three suggestions are much more than unlikely. Item D is likely.

References

Alexandridis, E. (1985) *The Pupil*, Springer, New York, pp. 56–67
Eskridge, J.B. *et al.* (1991) *Clinical Procedures in Optometry*, Lippincott, Philadelphia, p. 416
Hart, W.M. (ed.) (1992) *Adler's Physiology of the Eye*, 9th edn, Mosby, St Louis, pp. 434–439
Newman, N.M. (1992) *Neuro-ophthalmology, a Practical Text*, Appleton & Lange, Norwalk, Connecticut, pp. 250–251
Roy, F.H. (1989) *Ocular Syndromes and Systemic Diseases*, 2nd edn, Saunders, Philadelphia, pp. 12 and 205
Snell, R.S. and Lemp, M.A. (1989) *Clinical Anatomy of the Eye*, Blackwell Scientific, Boston, pp. 316–317
Spalton, D.J. *et al.* (1984) *Atlas of Clinical Ophthalmology*, Churchill Livingstone, Edinburgh, pp. 19.16 and 2.7

9 Item A is correct. The side effects of the eye drops may include a lowered heart rate. The effect of the drug is to decrease aqueous production.

References

Bartlett, J.D. and Jaanus, S.D. (1989) *Clinical Ocular Pharmacology*, 2nd edn, Butterworths, Boston, pp. 93–100
Berggren, L. (1990) Pharmacological and clinical aspects of glaucoma therapy. *Acta Ophthalmologica*, **68**, 497–507
Krupin, T. (1988) *Manual of Glaucoma Diagnosis and Management*, Churchill Livingstone, New York, p. 124
Wax, M. (1992) In *Pharmacology of Glaucoma* (eds S.M. Drance *et al.*), Williams & Wilkins, Baltimore, pp. 110 and 190–191

10 Both A and B appear to have some credibility, but the other suggestions do not.

References

Abraham, S.V. (1966) Control of myopia with tropicamide. *J Pediat Ophthalmol*, **3**, 10–22
Jensen, H. and Goldschmidt, E. (1991) In *Refractive Anomalies* (eds T. Grosvenor and M.C. Flom), Butterworth-Heinemann, pp. 371–383
Obata, S. (1944) Pilocarpine cure of myopia and pseudomyopia. *Acta Soc Ophthalmol Japan*, **48**, p. 241 (relates to item A)
Sampson, W.G. (1979) Role of cycloplegia in the management of functional myopia. *Ophthalmology*, **86**, 695–697
Stewart-Black Kelly, B. *et al.* (1975) Clinical assessment of the arrest of myopia. *Br J Ophthalmol*, **59**, 529–538 (particularly related to item C)

11 A common enquiry when a patient is having an eye examination seeks information about any drugs or prescribed medication which the patient is taking. This is chiefly in order to anticipate any possible ocular side effects. Which of the following suggestions is most likely *not* to be correct?

   A   Ergotamine tartrate or similar substances are often used in the treatment of migraine

   B   Diuretic drugs are used in several conditions, for instance hypertension; initially they may cause transient myopia and over a long time can reduce intraocular pressure

   C   Prescribed angiotensin converting enzyme (ACE) inhibitors, presumed to inhibit production of angiotensive substances, are unlikely to have been given with a view to reducing high blood pressure

   D   Amphetamines or some travel sickness antidotes may cause mydriasis and decrease the response of the pupils to light

12 Various medications are prescribed for patients for use directly on the eyes. Other medications have side effects upon the eyes or on ocular function. Which of the following is most likely to be correct?

   A   Beta-blockers which may reduce the production of aqueous humour are likely to produce a significant miosis, which will influence the outflow of aqueous

   B   The administration of pilocarpine hydrochloride 2 per cent into the conjunctival sac of a normal eye, three times a day, will greatly lower the intraocular pressure

   C   The application of a drug such as pilocarpine by an ocular insert placed in the conjunctival sac (even when maintained in place) is unreliable and ensures high systemic absorption

   D   A sympathomimetic agent, 1 per cent adrenaline, dropped into the conjunctival sac, probably reduces aqueous humour production by an influence on beta receptors, but also tends to increase outflow by affecting alpha receptors

   E   The pulsative ocular blood flow, probably a good measure of the ciliary–choroidal circulation, does not react differently to different beta-blockers over a long period

Drug uses and actions for optometrists: Answers

11 Item C, alone, is incorrect, since ACE inhibitors are now often used in the treatment of hypertension. There are insignificant ocular side effects in most cases, but headache is one possibility.

References

Bartlett, J.D. and Jaanus, S.D. (1989) *Clinical Ocular Pharmacology*, 2nd edn, Butterworths, Boston, pp. 814–817

Rosenbloom, A.A. and Morgan, M.W. (1993) *Vision and Aging*, 2nd edn, Butterworth-Heinemann, Boston, p. 165

Saper, J.R. (1987) (ed.) *Controversies and Clinical Variants of Migraine*, Pergamon, New York, pp. 4 and 99

Strube, G. and Strube, G. (1992) *ACE Inhibitors in Hypertension*, Kluwer Academic, Dordrecht, pp. 55 and 70

12 Item D should be chosen as being correct, while the other items are misleading.

References

Berggren, L. (1990) Pharmacological and clinical aspects of glaucoma therapy. *Acta Ophthalmol*, **68**, 497–507

Carenini, A.B. *et al.* (1994) Differences in the longterm effect of timolol and betaxolol on the pulsative ocular blood flow. *Surv Ophthalmol*, **38**, S118–S124

Hopkins, S.J. (1993) The drug treatment of glaucoma. *Optometry Today*, **33**, 24–26

Nyman, K. (1993) Intraocular pressure reduction with topically administered pilocarpine, timolol and betaxolol in normal tension glaucoma. *Acta Ophthalmol*, **71**, 686–690

13 Angle closure (in patients over 30 years of age) resulting from use of a mydriatic is likely to occur in approximately:

A   1 in 50 patients
B   1 in 500 patients
C   1 in 5000 patients
D   1 in 50 000 patients

14 Prior to instillation of mydriatics, it is wise to ensure that the anterior chamber has a minimum depth (at the centre of the cornea) of:

A   1.5 mm
B   2.0 mm
C   2.5 mm
D   3.0 mm
E   3.5 mm

15 Which of the following may legally be obtained by and then supplied by a British optometrist for use by the patient?

A   Amethocaine hydrochloride
B   Framycetin sulphate
C   Oxyphenbutazone eye ointment
D   Pilocarpine hydrochloride

16 Thiomersal is commonly used as a preservative in contact lens solutions, and in eye drops. Which of the following is *incorrect*?

A   Solutions containing this compound should be protected from light
B   Rubber caps remove thiomersal from the solution
C   Thiomersal is more stable in acid solutions (pH 7 to 9)
D   Bactericidal effect is due to the release of mercurial ions

17 Which ocular surface is the principal absorber of drugs instilled for therapeutic effect to the eye?

A   Cornea
B   Bulbar conjunctiva
C   Palpebral conjunctiva

Drug uses and actions for optometrists: Answers

13 D is correct.

References
Keller, J.T. (1975) The risk of angle closure from the use of mydriatics. *J Am Optom Assoc*, **46**, 19–21

Townsend, J.C. (1991) Anterior chamber angle estimation. In *Clinical Procedures in Optometry* (eds J.B. Eskridge), Lippincott, Philadelphia, pp. 36–38

14 C is correct.

References
Aizawa, K. (1958) The depth of the normal anterior chamber. *Acta Soc Ophthalmol Jpn*, **62**, 2283–2294

Borish, I.M. (1970) *Clinical Refraction*, 3rd edn, Professional Press, Chicago, p. 452

Townsend, J.C. (1991) Anterior chamber angle estimation. In *Clinical Procedures in Optometry* (eds J.B. Eskridge, J.F. Amos and J.D. Bartlett), Lippincott, Philadelphia, pp. 36–38

15 D is the only one that may be supplied to the patient; the others may be used by the optometrist, but may not be supplied to the patient.

Reference
British College of Optometrists (1994) *Optometrist's Formulary*, No. 2, London, pp. 4–7

16 C is incorrect; thiomersal is most stable in alkaline solutions pH 5 to 7.

Reference
O'Connor Davies, P.H. (1981) *The Actions and Uses of Ophthalmic Drugs*, 2nd edn, pp. 251–252, Butterworths, London

17 A is the correct response; both the ocular and palpebral conjunctiva absorb drugs instilled into the eye. However, much of the drug then enters the systemic circulation and is thus lost to the eye.

Reference
Vale, J. and Cox, B. (1985) *Drugs and the Eye*, 2nd edn, Butteworths, London, pp. 17–19

18 Which of the following adverse effects are unlikely to be caused by the use of anticholinesterase drugs (used in the treatment of myasthenia gravis)?

A Miosis
B Mydriasis
C Diplopia
D Lacrimation

19 Miotics can be used to reverse the effect of a mydriatic; however, the miotic must be chosen according to the mydriatic used. Following the use of tropicamide, which of the following miotics would *not* be appropriate?

A Physostigmine
B Pilocarpine
C Thymoxamine

20 When would atropine be used instead of occlusion therapy?

A In a non-cooperative patient whose amblyopic eye has visual acuity of 6/24 or better
B In a non-cooperative patient whose amblyopic eye has visual acuity of 6/24 or worse
C In a non-cooperative patient whose better eye has visual acuity of 6/24 or worse
D In a cooperative patient whose amblyopic eye has visual acuity of 6/24 or better

Drug uses and actions for optometrists: Answers

18 B is correct. Anticholinesterase drugs, as used in the diagnosis and treatment of myasthenia gravis tend to cause miosis, reduced VA, diplopia and lacrimation.

Reference

O'Connor Davies, P.H. (1981). *The Actions and Uses of Ophthalmic Drugs.* 2nd edn, Butterworths, London. p. 355.

19 C is correct. Tropicamide is a muscarinic antagonist and as such requires the use of muscarinic agonists such as pilocarpine and physostigmine to achieve reversal. Thymoxamine is a sympathetic antagonist which competes with sympathetic agonists such as phenylephrine for the α-receptors.

Reference

Vale, J. (1988). In *Optometry*, (eds K. Edwards and R. Llewelyn). Butterworths, London. p. 445.

20 A is correct. In this technique the child requires reasonable acuity in the amblyopic eye as he will be using this eye for reading and close work. There are several disadvantages, for example the risk of inducing allergies, hallucination, and, as it takes 1–2 weeks to wear off, there is the possibility of stimulus deprivation amblyopia in a young child. It is for this last reason that one would usually choose patching over atropine, making D an incorrect response.

Reference

Mein, J. and Harcourt, B. (1986). *Diagnosis and Management of Ocular Motility Disorders*. Blackwell Scientific, Oxford. pp. 184–185.